BY ANASTASIA MYSHUK

MW00954138

# *About the Author*

Anastasia Myshuk is a skilled nurse with years of experience in critical care, surgery, and cardiology. Her book, Hassle Free Anti-Inflammatory Diet, is a testament to her passion for health and wellness and her profound medical knowledge. Throughout her career, Anastasia has recognized food's vital role as medicine, particularly in reducing and preventing inflammation that can lead to chronic diseases. This realization sparked her love for cooking, inspiring her to create meals that are delicious and packed with anti-aging ingredients and brain-boosting foods, all aimed at promoting a longer, healthier life.

Born near the northern shores of the Black Sea and raised in a sun-drenched Mediterranean-like environment, Anastasia enjoyed fresh, wholesome foods. Her exposure to diverse cuisines fueled her passion for cooking. Over the years, she has infused her culinary love with healthy twists, blending family recipes from her childhood to create vibrant, nourishing meals.

This foundation of knowledge and creativity is the essence of Anastasia's new Hustle-Free Anti-Inflammatory Diet Cookbook. She shares quick and easy recipes in this collection, including a version inspired by Dr. Axe Healing Foods Diet, tailored for busy families and individuals. Her practical approach makes healthy eating accessible and enjoyable for novice and experienced cooks alike.

Balancing her roles as a mother of two, a frequent traveler, and a dedicated professional, Anastasia draws from her extensive travels to incorporate global flavors into her cooking. She shares her love of cooking and wellness in her book, offering delicious, easy-to-prepare, weight-friendly, and anti-inflammatory meals.

# Table of Contents

# Table of Contents

# Table of Contents

# Table of Contents

**CHAPTER #5**
**Meal Planning And Advanced Prep Techniques**

# Table of Contents

# 60-DAY MEAL PLAN

# GROCERY LIST

# INTRODUCTION

Jean Anthelme Brillat-Savarin once said, "Tell me what you eat, and I will tell you what you are."

Like many of us, I considered the purpose of food to be to satisfy our hunger and to give us the satiety to perform our daily chores comfortably. However, as life unfolded, I realized that food is more than a tool to feed our hunger. It is a powerful way to shape our health, well-being, and lives.

My name is Anastasia, and I live in the United States with my two kids. Like many other on-the-go moms, I used to believe that food was just fuel that ran our bodies. It might be something you grabbed on the go, often from a fast-food spot or a convenience store shelf. I was busy and always on the run, juggling school, work, and social life. I never had enough time to think about what I was putting into my body. I was eating sugary cereals, processed products, fast food, and sodas to keep me going. It was all about convenience, and I did not think twice about the long list of ingredients or the nutrition labels. I could keep up this pace for a while.

However, with time, things started to change. I began feeling lethargic all the time, no matter how much sleep I got. Once clear and glowing, my skin became dull and prone to acne and zits. I started feeling frequent stomach aches and digestion problems. My concentration span got shorter, my memory was slipping, and my mood swings were all over the place.

I thought it was due to my stress and busy lifestyle. Nevertheless, as the symptoms worsened, I realized something was wrong with my health. I was constantly bloated, and my energy levels were low all the time. Even the simplest tasks felt overwhelming. I did not feel like myself anymore, and it was scary. I was constantly pondering what had happened to my health and body. What did I do wrong? And what could I do to improve things?

One day, after another fast-food meal left me feeling bloated, I decided to examine my diet. I started researching and was astonished by the information about the negative impact of fast foods and the importance of an anti-inflammatory diet. I had been feeding my body nothing but junk, and frankly, I was feeling like junk. This is when I decided to redesign my dietary choices and restore my health. I was determined to change my eating habits and stop eating processed and sugary foods. I wanted to replace these food items with fresh fruits, vegetables, pulses such as beans and lentils, whole cereal products, and juices.

I checked my blood glucose level, which fluctuated often. The food I ate also compromised my cardiovascular health. My previous dietary choices included foods rich in saturated fats, sugars, and salt. These harmful ingredients increase the fatty tissues inside your body and make you vulnerable not only to obesity but also heart issues, insulin resistance, and eventually diabetes.

# INTRODUCTION

I started learning how to read food labels and which ingredients benefit my health. My journey led me to discover the power of anti-inflammatory foods that help reduce my risk of chronic inflammatory disease. It was tough initially. I had to break long-standing habits and rethink everything I knew about food. However, the results were almost immediate. I regained my energy levels, my brain fog lifted, and my skin cleared up. My digestion issues were solved, and those constant stomach aches disappeared.

The most surprising part was how much I began to enjoy cooking and experimenting with new anti-inflammatory recipes. I discovered the healing power of anti-inflammatory foods like turmeric, ginger, and leafy greens. I felt more connected to my eating, and my body responded positively. The change was not just physical but also mental and emotional. I felt empowered knowing I had taken control of my health and well-being.

Now, I cannot imagine going back to my previous dietary routine. My journey has taught me that food is more than just fuel—it is medicine, nourishment, and a way to care for you most fundamentally. I am not perfect, and still indulge now and then, but I have learned the importance of balance. The difference is that now, I am in control and know how to listen to my body. Healthy eating has become my preferred lifestyle.

I have learned through this journey that the choices we make every day matter. Grabbing a bag of chips instead of an apple might seem small, but those choices increase the risk of developing various chronic illnesses over time. I am living proof that it is never too late to make a change, and I hope my story can inspire others to take that first step toward a healthier, happier life.
It is not just about avoiding illness; it is about thriving, about living your best life. In addition, it all starts with what is on your plate.

**Let's take the first step towards changing your life!**

# CHAPTER 1

## GET STARTED WITH ANTI-INFLAMMATORY EATING

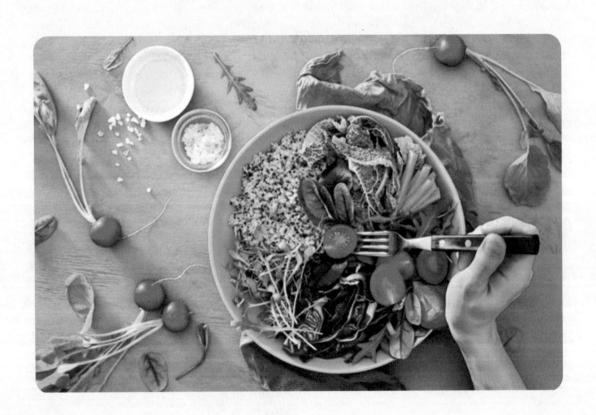

# Understanding inflammation and your body

Inflammation is our body's natural defensive mechanism that protects us from various chronic health conditions. It works like the "body's internal alarm system" that warms our immune system when there is an injury or infection inside the body. Inflammation works only when it is a short-term response, and it becomes harmful if it stays longer than expected. Then it is called chronic inflammatory response, which might trigger serious health problems like diabetes, inflammatory bowel disease, liver disease, and cardiovascular disorders. In this chapter, you will explore what inflammation is, how it influences your body, and how your diet can affect it. These basic concepts will help you to make informed choices to support your health and well-being.

## What is inflammation?

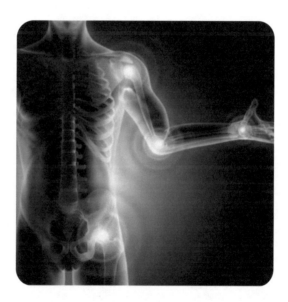

It is known as a biological and chemical response to injury or infection. Your body starts an inflammatory process when it detects any threat, such as a cut, toxin invasion, or disease, inside the body. The body activates your immune system to repair itself by initiating a chain of mechanisms. Inflammatory mechanisms involve releasing many chemicals and immune cells that work to remove or neutralize the threat and cure the affected area. Four cardinal signs of inflammation include redness, swelling, heat, and pain.

## Mechanism of inflammation

When we talk about the mechanism behind the inflammatory processes, there are two forms of inflammation, which involve separate biological mechanisms. These two forms are acute inflammation and chronic inflammation. Acute inflammation, as a short-term response, occurs immediately after an infection, injury, or toxin invasion. For instance, a wound on your hand becomes swollen, red, hot, or warm. Moreover, you will feel pain in that affected area. It is acute inflammation at work. White blood cells in your body get activated in this situation and rush toward the sight of infection to fight off any pathogen. This short-term response is generally beneficial and mandatory for healing. Once the damage is recovered, acute inflammation settles, and your body returns to normal.

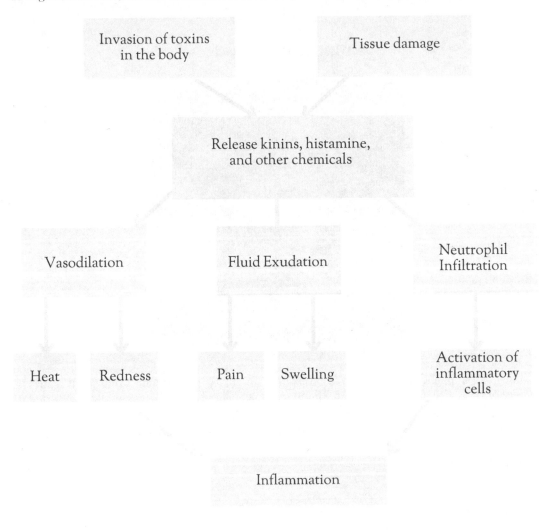

Inflammation becomes chronic and prolonged if it lasts for months or even years. Chronic inflammation continues even when there is no immediate danger because it does not resolve after the threat is gone. This prolonged effect can be due to persistent body infections, autoimmune disorders, or unhealthy lifestyle choices (including poor dietary choices and a sedentary routine). Arthritis, an autoimmune disease of joints, is an example of chronic inflammation in which your immune system mistakenly attacks your joints, causing pain and swelling.

Obesity is another example of a chronic inflammatory response in which excess fatty tissues release inflammatory chemicals. These inflammatory chemicals can lead to various health issues, including diabetes and cardiovascular diseases.

## Acute vs. Chronic Inflammation

| Acute Inflammation | Chronic Inflammation |
|---|---|
| Short term response | Long term response |
| Causes flushed skin at the site of the injury, pain or tenderness, swelling, and heat | Causes abdominal pain, chest pain, fever, mouth sores, fatigue or insomnia, joint pain or stiffness, depression & anxiety, weight gain or weight loss, acid reflux, diarrhea, and frequent infections |
| Inflammatory cells travel to the site of injury or infection and start the healing process | The body continues sending inflammatory cells even when there's no danger |
| Example: strep throat, enteritis | Example: rheumatoid arthritis |

## Diet and inflammation

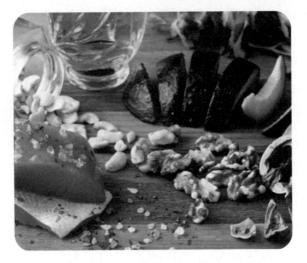

Diet has a direct link to inducing or eradicating inflammation in your body. Certain foods are pro-inflammatory because they cause inflammation. On the other hand, certain foods have anti-inflammatory potential because they reduce inflammatory responses in your body and help maintain your overall health. Therefore, it is vital to understand the nature of the food you consume to help make better dietary choices depending on your current health status.

### Pro-inflammatory foods

These foods worsen inflammation by triggering the inflammatory mechanism. pro-inflammatory foods are rich in refined sugars, processed ingredients, and trans fats. Most snack foods you consume daily (e.g., candies, soft drinks sodas, and bakery items) trigger inflammation. These foods cause spikes in blood glucose levels, leading to an inflammatory response. Moreover, processed products, including fast foods and packaged snacks, are great sources of trans fats and additives that can promote inflammation. Therefore, be careful when you consume these food items if you are already at risk of any chronic inflammatory health condition.

A research study published in The Journal of Clinical Endocrinology & Metabolism concluded that increased sugar consumption is associated with a raised level of inflammatory markers in the body. Similar research published in The American Journal of Clinical Nutrition concluded that trans-fat consumption is linked with higher levels of inflammatory markers.

### Anti-inflammatory foods

Certain fruits, vegetables, whole grain products, and omega-3-rich foods are anti-inflammatory because these foods help reduce inflammation. Fruits like berries, vegetables like leafy greens, dried fruits, and nuts are rich sources of omega-3 fatty acids, fiber, vitamins and minerals, and antioxidants. The Journal of Nutrition published a study concluding that increased fruit and vegetable consumption lowers inflammatory markers. A similar study has been published by The New England Journal of Medicine, which showed that omega-3-rich foods (including fish oil) reduce inflammation and lower the risk of chronic diseases.

**Symptoms of chronic inflammation**

The chronic inflammatory response is primarily asymptomatic at the initial stages. Symptoms are not obvious, so you are unaware of the damage it is causing to your body. However, with time, it becomes dangerous as it leads to several severe health conditions. Identifying the particular signs of inflammation and understanding the potential long-term effects can assist you in taking proactive measures to manage inflammation. Common symptoms of chronic inflammation include persistent fatigue, joint pain, and swelling.

# The basics of anti-inflammatory foods

Your diet can significantly reduce chronic inflammation. Choosing the right foods can help your body maintain a healthy balance, supporting overall well-being.

**Identifying anti-inflammatory foods**

Recently, the use of herbal plants has increased tremendously. People use them as therapeutic foods instead of medicines and drugs to prevent and treat chronic illnesses. These herbal plants contain various magical ingredients with antioxidant and anti-inflammatory potential. They are used to relieve chronic inflammation and oxidative stress.

If you consume fresh fruits and vegetables in your diet daily, you are consuming these magical ingredients as well because fruits and vegetables are rich sources of these ingredients, including vitamins, minerals, and phytochemicals. These foods prevent cellular stresses, inhibit inflammatory signals, promote healthy gut microbiota, and slow digestion. Antioxidants, omega-3 fatty acids, fiber, and other phytochemicals are some anti-inflammatory foods.

These foods reduce inflammation by balancing the blood glucose level, as elevated blood glucose can lead to insulin resistance and inflammation. Additionally, these magical foods maintain a balance between pathogens and healthy microorganisms in our gut, as dysbiosis negatively affects our immune system and eventually triggers inflammation.

**Following are some foods good to overcome inflammation:**

- Fatty fish: mackerel, salmon, and sardines are rich sources of omega-3 fatty acids
- Seeds and nuts: Chia seeds, almonds, and walnuts are rich in good fats and fiber
- Leafy green vegetables: these vegetables are rich in fiber, antioxidants, and other phytonutrients
- Berries: berries contain vitamins, antioxidants, and other active anti-inflammatory agents
- Olive oil: it is a good source of mono-unsaturated fatty acids and antioxidants

**Foods to avoid**

Many foods promote inflammation in the body. Excessive consumption of sugar, high fructose corn syrup, refined carbohydrates, and processed foods triggers inflammation by incorporating elevated blood glucose levels, insulin resistance, and fatty liver. Moreover, sugar, refined carbohydrates, and processed foods are poor in vital nutrients and disrupt the balance of bacteria in the gut, leading to inflammation. In addition, these foods generate free radicals inside our bodies and increase oxidative stress. Oxidative stress causes cellular damage, including cell membrane disruption, DNA damage, and chronic inflammation.

Earlier, we coined the term "pro-inflammatory foods." What do these foods do? These foods promote inflammatory reactions inside the body. For example, saturated and trans fats, including too much omega-6, are pro-inflammatory. If you consume these food items in excess daily, you will be at risk of coronary heart disease. Similarly, corn and soybean oil promote oxidative stress and inflammation when consumed excessively.

**Balancing a diet for optimal health**

What is a balanced diet? Do you think that the diet you consume daily is balanced?

If your answer is NO, no worries

We bring all the suitable answers for you.

A balanced diet is a diet that contains all the essential nutrients (macro and micronutrients) in the recommended proportion. United States Department of Agriculture (USDA) coined the term "Food Guide Pyramid" in 1992 to indicate the hierarchical distribution of all five primary food groups according to proportion. These five food groups include cereals, fruits, vegetables, dairy, and meat. A balanced diet contains food items from all these five food groups in recommended amounts daily.

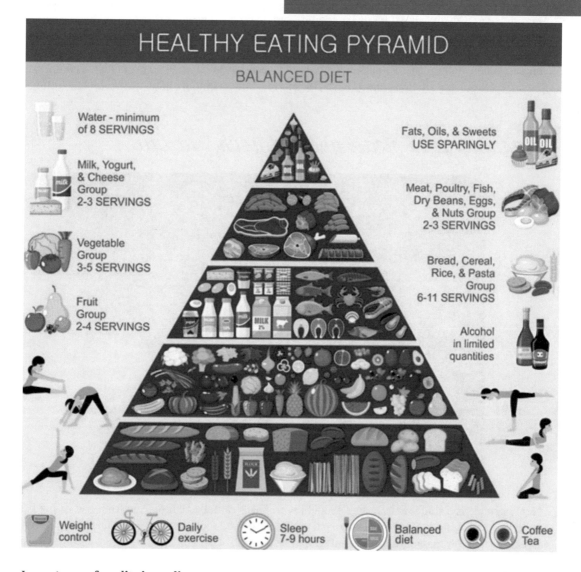

## HEALTHY EATING PYRAMID
### BALANCED DIET

Water - minimum of 8 SERVINGS

Milk, Yogurt, & Cheese Group 2-3 SERVINGS

Vegetable Group 3-5 SERVINGS

Fruit Group 2-4 SERVINGS

Fats, Oils, & Sweets USE SPARINGLY

Meat, Poultry, Fish, Dry Beans, Eggs, & Nuts Group 2-3 SERVINGS

Bread, Cereal, Rice, & Pasta Group 6-11 SERVINGS

Alcohol in limited quantities

Weight control | Daily exercise | Sleep 7-9 hours | Balanced diet | Coffee Tea

**Importance of quality ingredients**

It is mandatory to consume a balanced diet to achieve optimal health and minimize the risk of chronic illnesses. Macronutrients, including carbohydrates, proteins, and fats, are your body's building blocks and fuel your daily chores. Carbohydrate-rich food sources are cereals, rice, vegetables, and fruits. Carbohydrates give glucose to the blood, which is your body's primary fuel. You can get proteins from animal (meat) and plant (beans and pulses) sources. Protein is the vital building block of your body. Try to consume animal protein, which is more biologically available to your body. Fats include animal sources (meat) and plant sources (plant oils). Fats from the animals are saturated and unsuitable for human health if consumed in large amounts. Plant fat, such as olive oil, is unsaturated and good for brain health.

Micronutrients, including vitamins, minerals, and phytochemicals, are essential for various body functions, including muscle stretching, neural coordination, reproduction, and other vital involuntary chores. Vitamins are categorized as fat-soluble vitamins (A, D, E, & K) and water-soluble vitamins (B-complex and vitamin C). Water-soluble vitamins are essential in energy metabolism processes. Similarly, fat-soluble vitamins play crucial roles in the body, including bone health, blood clotting, and vision.

# Planning your meals around your schedule

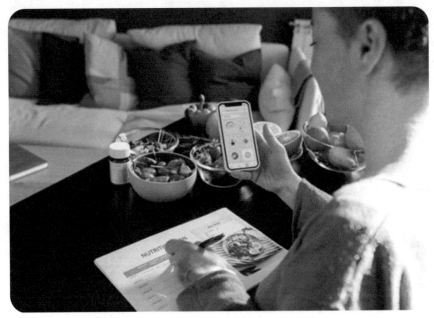

Meal planning is a skill that everyone should know. Meal planning relieves you from bad eating habits, including munching, random snacking, and eating processed foods at significant mealtimes. It plans a weekly or monthly menu to suit your nutritional needs best.

**Meal planning basics**

Following are the five basic steps for meal planning:
1. The first step is to determine your meal preparation technique according to your work routine and timings.
2. Once you have selected the preparation technique, pick a day of the week to prepare the menu for the week.
3. It is preferable to cook meals that you enjoy eating.
4. Make your shopping list for the whole week as it gives you the freedom of choosing something to eat on the spot (at significant mealtimes such as lunch).
5. Start with the small meals, easy recipes, convenient cooking techniques. Small steps lead to big results.

**Customized meal plan templates and time-saving**

Planning a meal for a week will be very easy if you already have meal-planning templates. With some basic knowledge, you can easily create customized meal plan templates. You should know the foods you like, readily available and affordable foods, and foods that contain all the essential nutrients to obtain optimal health and well-being.

Make colorful meal plan templates and paste them into your kitchen. It will give you a pleasant feeling that you put effort into improving your health and you care for yourself.

Moreover, it will save you time when deciding what to cook today. You already have a list of things to prepare for food daily. You only need to have a glance at your template in your kitchen and start making it without wasting time.

**Integrating new habits**

It is an ideal way to build healthy eating habits and a good lifestyle. Healthy eating habits will help you avoid eating processed and junk food, which ultimately will lead to bad health. Meal planning integrates the habit of giving time to yourself. You will spend some time in the week pondering the food choices that will make you healthy and fit. You will think about particular foods and their health benefits. You will research the impact of those foods on your body.

## Shopping smart: What to buy and what to avoid

Grocery shopping can be daunting; you may become sick of it if you have not planned. For example, if you want to shop for anti-inflammatory foods, research them and make a list before shopping. Advertisements, discounts on unhealthy foods, and eye-catching packaging can confuse you.

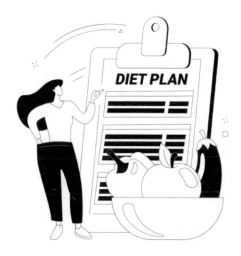

**Creating a Master Grocery List**

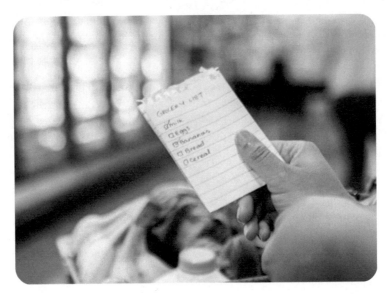

The best way to streamline your grocery shopping and avoid unnecessary purchases is to create a master grocery list. It is your go-to guide for every grocery store trip based on your body's nutritional needs. Start by planning your meals for the week. It does not have to be complicated; decide on a few breakfasts, lunches, dinners, and snacks. After that, list all the ingredients you will need. It could be the best option to keep you focused on your shopping goals.

**Seasonal Shopping**

Purchasing seasonal foods is a smart choice for cost savings and nutritional value. Seasonal fruits and vegetables are often fresher, tastier, and more nutrient-rich because they are harvested at their peak. They are also usually less expensive because they are more abundant.

In summer, you can purchase fresh berries, tomatoes, zucchini, and sweet potatoes, carrots, and beets which are available in winter. In this way, you will get better quality foods in a greater variety throughout the year.

**Decoding Marketing Tactics**

Marketing is a significant tool for increasing food product purchases at grocery stores. They use different advertising tools and tactics, from strategically placed snacks on the front shelf to limited-time discount offers on unhealthy food items. Therefore, you need to be careful and aware to outsmart these tricks.

Do not be attracted to flashy packaging and health claims, such as low fat, zero sugar, and no salt foods. These misleading information chunks might distract you and make you fall for the product. Try to learn how to read food labels and which nutrients benefit your health.

**Budgeting Tips**

Eating a healthy diet is not expensive. A few dietary strategies can help maintain a nutritious anti-inflammatory diet without overspending. To purchase food in bulk, like whole grains, nuts, seeds, and beans, you must have proper storage space and conditions like temperature and humidity checks. Purchasing food items in bulk can reduce the purchase amount of these products.

# Preparing your kitchen for success

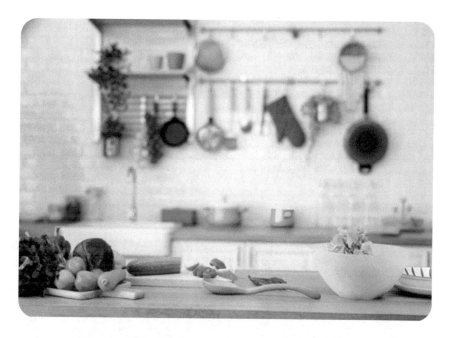

Your kitchen is the most precious spot in your home as it is directly linked to your health and well-being. This space must be up for success in maintaining a healthy anti-inflammatory diet. A well-organized and clean kitchen can make all the difference in sticking to your dietary goals and making meal prep an enjoyable experience.

**Setting up the Physical Space**

Kitchen layout significantly impacts how easily and efficiently you prepare your planned meals. It includes moving around your kitchen and setting the places for different food items, including spices. Your counter space must be clear and ready for action whenever needed.

It is helpful to organize your kitchen into small zones to store different things based on their use. For example, create a preparation zone near the sink and cutting boards to wash, chop, and prepare ingredients. A storage zone for dry and non-perishable goods helps to keep them safe. Organizing your kitchen will streamline your cooking process, making preparing healthy, anti-inflammatory meals quicker and more enjoyable.

### Stocking up on Essentials

A successful kitchen is well-stocked with the right tools and ingredients. You don't need every gadget on the market but having a few essential items can make a big difference in your cooking experience. Start with the basics: sharp knives, cutting boards, a good set of pots and pans, and some quality storage containers. These tools will be the foundation for most meal prep and cooking activities. Additionally, consider investing in a blender or food processor to make smoothies, sauces, and soups, often staples in an anti-inflammatory diet.

### Maintaining Cleanliness and Order

A clean and orderly kitchen makes cooking more pleasant and promotes better health by preventing cross-contamination and food-borne illnesses. Start by keeping your countertops clear and wiping them down regularly. Store ingredients in labeled containers and organize them in your pantry and fridge. It makes it easier to find what you need and reduces the chances of wasting food. Cleaning as you go is another habit that can make a huge difference.

### Encouraging a Positive Mindset

A well-organized, clean, and inviting kitchen can create a positive mindset around cooking and eating. Consider adding personal touches that make the space feel more welcoming, including a few plants, colorful dishware, or even a playlist of your favorite music while cooking. These small details can transform your kitchen from a functional space into a place you enjoy spending time in. When your kitchen is set up for success, staying motivated and committed to your health goals is more accessible.

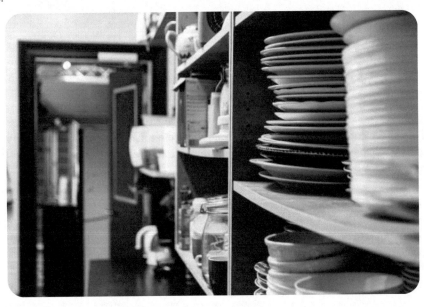

# CHAPTER 2

## SIMPLE AND QUICK RECIPES

### Five ingredients or fewer recipes

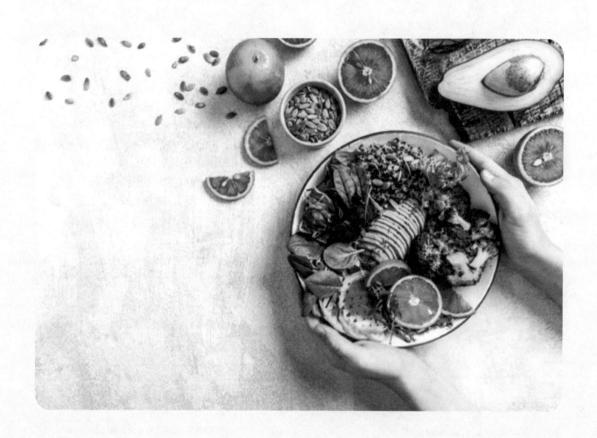

# 1. Mint Berry Fusion Smoothie:

Prep Time: 7 min l Cook Time: 0 min l Total Time: 10 min l Difficulty: Easy

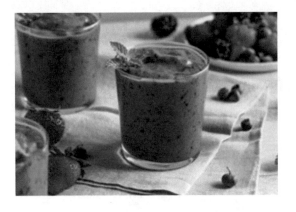

## Ingredients:

- ½ cup frozen mixed berries
- ¼ cup fresh mint leaves
- ½ cup unsweetened almond milk
- ¼ cup Plain Greek Yogurt
- 1 tsp flax seeds

## Instructions:

1. Blend all the ingredients until you get a smooth and creamy consistency.
2. Serve the smoothie in a glass and garnish it with mint leaves!

Total calories: 101 | Carbohydrates: 12g | Proteins: 8g | Fats:3g

# 2. Cinnamon & Ginger Infused Water:

Prep Time: 5 min l Cook Time: 5 min l Total Time: 10 min l Difficulty: Easy

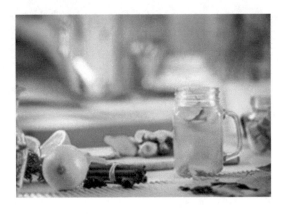

## Ingredients:

- 1.5 cup spring water
- 1-inch piece of ginger, peeled and grated
- ¼ tsp cinnamon
- one lemon or 1 tsp lemon juice

## Instructions:

1. Bring 1.5 cup water to a boil. Add ginger, cinnamon, and lemon juice and boil for 5-7 minutes.
2. Serve immediately and garnish with a slice of lemon on top!

Total calories: 9 | Carbohydrates: 2g | Proteins: 0g | Fats:0g

## 3. Paprika Roasted Cauliflower

Prep Time: 10 min l Cook Time: 20 min l Total Time: 30 min l Difficulty: Medium

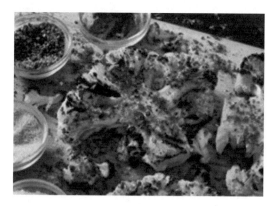

### Ingredients:

- 1 cup cauliflower florets
- 1 tbsp extra virgin olive oil
- 1 tsp smoked paprika
- Salt and pepper to taste

### Instructions:

1. Preheat your oven to 200 C.
2. Add cauliflower florets to a bowl, season them with smoked paprika, salt, pepper, and garlic powder, and mix well.
3. Grease a baking tray with 1 tbsp olive oil and spread the florets thoroughly. Roast them for about 20-25 minutes or until the cauliflower is golden and crispy.
4. Serve immediately.

Total calories: 154 | Carbohydrates: 6g | Proteins: 3g | Fats:14g

## 4. Turmeric & Fennel seed Tea

Prep Time: 5 min l Cook Time: 5 min l Total Time: 10 min l Difficulty: Easy

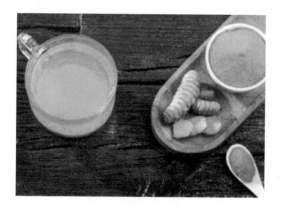

### Ingredients:

- 1.5 cup spring water
- ¼ tsp turmeric powder
- ½ tsp fennel seeds
- 1 tsp raw honey

### Instructions:

1. Bring 1.5 cups water to a boil. Add turmeric powder, fennel seeds, and ginger to the boiling water and boil for 5-7 minutes.
2. Serve immediately and garnish with a slice of lemon on top!

Total calories: 27 | Carbohydrates: 6g | Proteins: 0g | Fats:0g

## 5. Basil Cherry Refresher

Prep Time: 5 min l Cook Time: 0 min l Total Time: 10 min l Difficulty: Easy

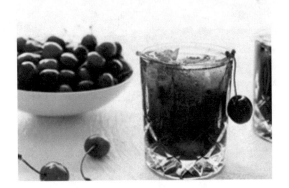

### Ingredients:

- ½ cup cherries, pitted
- 1 cup sparkling water or Coconut water
- 4-5 Fresh Basil leaves
- one lemon or 1 tsp lemon juice
- ¼ cup ice cubes

### Instructions:

1. Blend all ingredients in a blender at high speed.
2. Pour into a glass and garnish it with cherries on top!

Total calories: 4 | Carbohydrates: 1g | Proteins: 0g | Fats:0g

## 6. Roasted Brussels Sprouts and Pecans Salad

Prep Time: 10 min l Cook Time: 5 mins l Total Time: 15 min l Difficulty: Easy

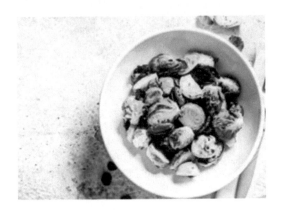

### Ingredients:

- 1 cup Brussels sprouts, halved and sauteed for 2-3 mins
- 5g pecans
- One lemon or 1 tbsp lemon juice
- 1 tsp Extra Virgin olive oil
- 1 tsp black pepper

### Instructions:

1. Sauté halved Brussels sprouts in one teaspoon of extra virgin olive oil for about 2-3 mins.
2. Combine all ingredients in a bowl. Add lemon juice and black pepper. Mix it well.
3. Serve immediately.

Total calories: 139 | Carbohydrates: 14g | Proteins: 5g | Fats:9g

# 7. Roasted Bok choy with garlic

## 8. Ginger and Mint Infused Green Tea

Prep Time: 5 min l Cook Time: 15 mins l Total Time: 20 min l Difficulty: Easy

Prep Time: 5 min l Cook Time: 5 mins l Total Time: 10 min l Difficulty: Easy

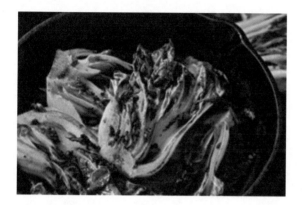

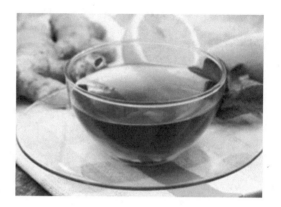

### Ingredients:

- One head of Baby Bok Choy, chopped
- One teaspoon of sesame oil
- 1-2 cloves of garlic
- 1/8 teaspoon red chili powder
- Sea salt as per taste

### Instructions:

1. Preheat your oven to 200 C.
2. Finely cut baby Bok choy into equal pieces. Add them to a bowl. Season them with garlic, red chili powder, and sea salt.
3. Grease a baking tray with 1 tbsp sesame oil and thoroughly spread the seasoned baby Bok choy. Roast for 15-20 minutes or until tender and crispy.
4. Serve immediately.

### Ingredients:

- 1 cup hot water
- 1-inch piece of ginger, peeled and sliced
- Several fresh mint leaves
- 1 Green Tea bag
- 1 tsp manuka honey

### Instructions:

1. Boil one cup of water in a pan for 3-5 minutes on medium heat. Add ginger slices and fresh mint leaves.
2. Strain this into a cup, place a green tea bag, and let it rest for 3-5 minutes. Add one teaspoon of honey for a sweeter kick.
3. Serve immediately.

Total calories: 59 | Carbohydrates: 3.7g | Proteins: 1.4g | Fats:4.7g

Total calories: 27 | Carbohydrates: 1g | Proteins: 0g | Fats:0g

# 1. Ginger & Turmeric Carrot soup

Prep Time: 7-10 min l Cook Time: 7-10 mins l Total Time: 15-20 min l Difficulty: Easy

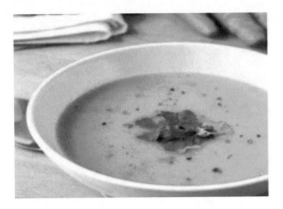

**Ingredients:**

- 2 cups carrot, peeled and chopped
- 1 cup of sodium vegetable broth
- A one-inch piece of ginger, peeled and grated
- ¼ teaspoon turmeric powder
- Two cloves of garlic, finely chopped
- Salt and pepper as per taste
- ½ small onion, peeled and chopped
- 1 tsp extra virgin olive oil
- 1 teaspoon parsley

**Instructions:**

1. Heat extra virgin olive in a pot over medium heat. Add chopped onion, grated ginger, garlic, carrots, and Sauté for 2 minutes.
2. Add vegetable broth and boil for 5-7 minutes or until carrots are tender.
3. Blend this mixture until it reaches a soup-like consistency, season with salt, pepper, and fresh parsley.
4. Serve while hot.

Total calories: 216 | Carbohydrates: 41g | Proteins: 4g | Fats:5g

# 2. Grilled Salmon and Cucumber Tortilla wrap

Prep Time: 7-10 min l Cook Time: 5-9 mins l Total Time: 15-20 min l Difficulty: Medium

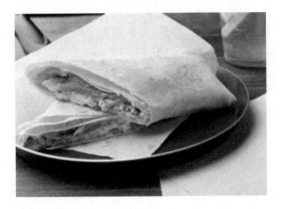

**Ingredients:**

- One small-sized salmon fillet (3-4 oz)
- One whole wheat tortilla wrap
- One small cucumber, sliced
- ½ cup cherry tomatoes, sliced

Salmon seasoning:
- Salt and pepper as per taste
- 1 tsp fresh dill or parsley
- Pinch of garlic powder

For the sauce:
- Three tablespoons of Greek yogurt
- 1 tbsp low-fat mayonnaise
- 1/8 tsp garlic powder
- Pinch of red chili flakes

**Instructions:**

1. Heat extra virgin olive in a Grill pan. Add seasoned salmon and grill for 3-4 minutes on each side.
2. Warm the tortilla wrap for 30 seconds on each side.
3. Spread the sauce evenly on the wrap. Add cucumber slices and salmon fillet to it. Fold it into a wrap and enjoy!

Total calories: 402 | Carbohydrates: 31g | Proteins: 4g | Fats:5g

## 3. Mixed Greens Avocado Salad

Prep Time: 15min | Cook Time: 0 mins | Total Time: 15 min | Difficulty: Easy

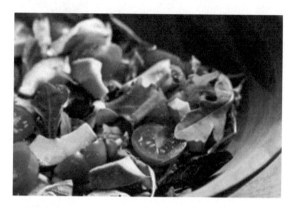

### Ingredients:

- Two cups mixed greens (Spinach, arugula, or lettuce), chopped
- ½ cup cherry tomatoes, sliced
- ½ small red onion, peeled and chopped
- 50g ripe avocado, sliced
- ¼ cup feta cheese
- 1 tbsp mixed nuts (optional for topping)

Salad dressing:
- 1 tsp extra virgin olive oil
- ½ tsp black pepper
- 1 tsp balsamic vinegar
- 1 tsp tzatziki sauce

### Instructions:

1. Place the chopped mixed greens and avocado in a bowl. Drizzle the salad dressing and toss until well combined.
2. Add feta cheese and mixed nuts to make this salad tastier and crunchier.

Total calories: 420 | Carbohydrates: 47g | Proteins: 22g | Fats:39g

## 4. Chickpea Lettuce Salad Jar

Prep Time: 15 min | Cook Time: 0 min | Total Time: 15 min | Difficulty: Easy

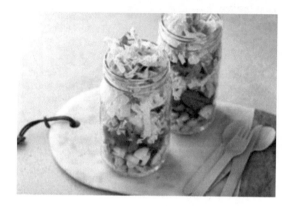

### Ingredients:

- ½ cup canned chickpeas
- ½ cup cherry tomatoes, sliced
- 1 cup lettuce, chopped
- ¼ cup cucumber, chopped
- ¼ cup bell peppers, diced

For Salad Dressing:
- 1 tsp extra virgin olive oil
- Sea salt and pepper as per taste
- 1 tsp lemon juice
- 1 tsp oregano or parsley

### Instructions:

1. Mix extra virgin olive oil, salt, pepper, lemon juice, and oregano in a small bowl.
2. In a jar, add this dressing and layer it with chickpeas, followed by cucumber, bell peppers, and cherry tomatoes.
3. Add Lettuce leaves on top and shake the jar to mix the dressing evenly.
4. Serve immediately.

Total calories:225 | Carbohydrates: 47g | Proteins: 9g | Fats:7g

# 5. Stir Fry Garlic Broccoli Rice

# 6. Spinach Mushroom Frittata with Parmesan Cheese

Prep Time: 5 min l Cook Time: 5 mins l Total Time: 10 min l Difficulty: Easy & Quick

Prep Time: 7 min l Cook Time: 4 mins l Total Time: 11 min l Difficulty: Easy

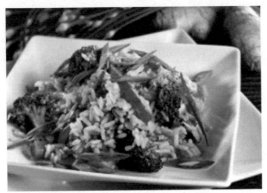

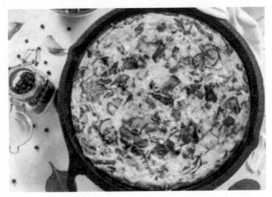

## Ingredients:

- 1 cup broccoli florets
- ½ small carrot, peeled and sliced
- ¼ cup bell pepper, diced
- 1-2 cloves of garlic, chopped
- one tablespoon soya sauce
- 1 tbsp oyster sauce
- one teaspoon of sesame oil
- ¼ teaspoon chili flakes
- one teaspoon of extra virgin olive oil
- ½ teaspoon sesame seeds (For garnish

## Instructions:

1. Heat olive oil in a medium-sized pan and sauté chopped garlic for 1 minute.
2. Add broccoli florets, sliced carrots, diced bell peppers, and stir-fry for 2-3 minutes on medium to high heat.
3. Add soy sauce, oyster sauce, chili flakes, and sesame oil, and stir fry again for 1 minute.
4. Add the boiled rice into this stir-fry mixture and toss them well.
5. Add sesame seeds on top and serve.

Total calories: 236 | Carbohydrates: 36g | Proteins: 6.7g | Fats: 9.7g

## Ingredients:

- Two medium eggs
- ¼ cup fresh baby spinach leaves, chopped
- ¼ cup mushrooms
- ¼ cup sliced bell peppers
- One tablespoon grated parmesan cheese
- Salt and pepper as per taste
- 1 tsp mixed herbs
- 1 teaspoon of olive oil

## Instructions:

1. Place a nonstick pan over medium heat. Grease it with olive oil.
2. Whisk the eggs in a bowl. Add baby spinach leaves, mushrooms, bell peppers, salt, pepper, mixed herbs, and parmesan cheese. Mix well.
3. Spread this mixture in a pan and cook for 3-4 minutes on each side until fully cooked.
4. Serve this frittata on a plate, cut it into squares, and pair it with whole-grain toast.

Total calories: 290 | Carbohydrates: 17g | Proteins: 23g | Fats:22g

## 7. Avocado hummus with stir fry veggies

Prep Time: 15 min l Cook Time: 0 mins l Total Time: 15 min l Difficulty: Easy

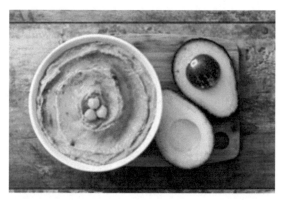

## 8. Peanut butter Toast with Berries

Prep Time: 7 min l Cook Time: 0 mins l Total Time: 7 min l Difficulty: Easy & Quick

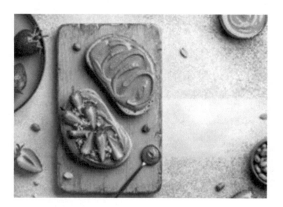

**Ingredients:**

- 1/2 cup canned chickpeas
- ½ ripe avocado, pitted and chopped
- 1 tsp lemon juice
- 1 tbsp Tahini
- 1/8 tsp garlic powder
- Salt and pepper as per taste
- 1 tbsp extra virgin olive oil
- Stir fry veggies:
- ½ small zucchini peeled and cut into long, thick slices
- ½ small carrot peeled and cut into long, thick slices

**Instructions:**

1. Place drained canned chickpeas, avocado, tahini, lemon juice, garlic powder, salt, pepper, and extra virgin olive oil in a food processor. Add a bit of water to make a smooth paste if required. Set it aside.
2. Sauté veggies in a pan greased with extra virgin olive oil for 3-4 minutes on medium heat until the crisp comes over them. Sprinkle a pinch of black pepper and thyme over.

Total calories: 520 | Carbwohydrates: 52g | Proteins: 11g | Fats:46g

**Ingredients:**

- One slice of whole-grain bread
- 2 tbsp of Peanut butter
- ¼ cup strawberries, sliced
- Pinch of cinnamon powder
- 1 tsp manuka honey (Optional)

**Instructions:**

1. Spread 1-2 tbsp Peanut butter evenly on a whole-grain bread slice. Layer sliced strawberries and sprinkle a pinch of cinnamon powder on top. Drizzle 1 tsp of manuka honey, if desired.
2. Serve immediately.

Total calories: 320 | Carbohydrates: 44g | Proteins: 15g | Fats: 20g

# 1. Mixed berries Chia Seed Pudding

Prep Time: 7min l Cook Time: 0 mins l Total Time: 4 hours l Difficulty: Easy

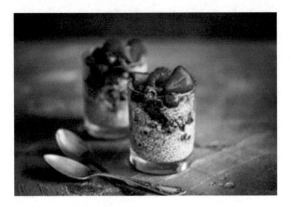

**Ingredients:**

- 2.5 tbsp chia seeds
- ½ cup almond milk or any plant-based milk
- 2 tbsp Plain Greek yogurt or almond yogurt
- ¼ tsp cinnamon powder
- 1 tsp raw honey
- ½ tsp vanilla extract
- For the Topping:
- 5g walnuts, crushed
- 5g almonds, crushed
- 5g Pecans, crushed
- ½ cup mixed berries (strawberries, raspberries, blueberries)

**Instructions:**

1. Add almond milk to a bowl, then chia seeds, plain Greek yogurt or almond yogurt, cinnamon powder, honey, and vanilla extract. Mix it well. Leave it overnight or for 3-4 hours in the fridge.
2. Top it with almonds, walnuts, pecans, and mixed berries.
3. Serve immediately.

Total calories: 420 | Carbohydrates: 77g | Proteins: 20g | Fats: 20g

# 2. Quinoa Mixed Veggie Breakfast Bowl

Prep Time: 10min l Cook Time: 25 mins l Total Time: 35 mins l Difficulty: Easy

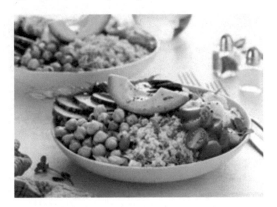

**Ingredients:**

- ½ cup quinoa
- 1 cup spring water
- ½ cup baby spinach, chopped
- ½ small zucchini, diced
- ½ cup cherry tomatoes
- 1 tbsp extra virgin olive oil
- Salt and pepper as per taste
- For topping:
- ¼ cup feta cheese
- ¼ avocado, pitted and sliced
- ¼ cup parsley

**Instructions:**

1. Cook the quinoa. Add the rinsed quinoa and spring water to a pan and boil on medium heat.
2. Let it cook for about 15-20 minutes. Set it aside.
3. Sauté mixed veggies (spinach, zucchini, cherry tomatoes) in a pan for 3-4 minutes. Sprinkle salt and pepper over them.
4. In a bowl, add cooked quinoa and place a layer of sauteed mixed veggies. Add the sliced avocado, feta cheese, and fresh parsley leaves.
5. Serve immediately.

Total calories: 520 | Carbohydrates: 60g | Proteins: 21g | Fats:44g

## 3. Ginger Pear Fusion Smoothie

## 4. Blueberry infused Greek Yogurt Parfait

Prep Time: 8 min l Cook Time: 0 mins l Total Time: 10 mins l Difficulty: Easy

Prep Time: 10 min l Cook Time: 10 mins l Total Time: 20 mins l Difficulty: Medium

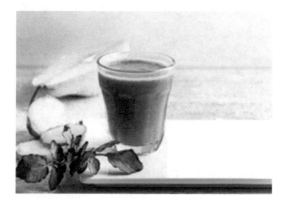

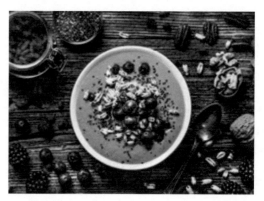

### Ingredients:

- one large ripe pear, chopped
- ½ small green apple, peeled and chopped
- 1 cup almond milk or soy milk
- ½ cup plain Greek yogurt
- 2 tbsp oats
- 5g cashews
- 1-inch piece of ginger peeled and grated
- 1 tsp acacia honey
- 1 tsp hemp seeds
- Ice cubes as needed

### Instructions:

1. Combine all ingredients in a blender. Blend at high speed until you achieve a smooth consistency.
2. Serve immediately.

### Ingredients:

- For the blueberry Puree:
- ½ cup fresh or frozen blueberries
- 1 Tbsp of honey
- For Parfait:
- 1 cup plain greek yogurt
- 1 tsp chia seeds soaked in water for 10-15 mins
- 2 tbsp granola
- 1 tbsp mixed nuts
- Few blueberries (for garnish)

### Instructions:

1. Add blueberries, honey, and a few drops of water to a saucepan and cook for 5-7 minutes until the mixture is pureed. Allow it to cool.
2. In a small bowl, add half of the Greek yogurt and blueberry puree. Then, add a layer of chia seeds over it.
3. Place the remaining layers of Greek yogurt, followed by blueberry puree.
4. Top it with mixed nuts, blueberries, and granola for an extra crunch.
5. Serve immediately.

Total calories: 425 | Carbohydrates: 95g | Proteins: 25g | Fats: 20g

Total calories: 400 | Carbohydrates: 72g | Proteins: 38g | Fats:10g

## 5. Apple Cinnamon Oatmeal with Mixed Nuts

Prep Time: 5 min l Cook Time: 10 mins l Total Time: 15 mins l Difficulty: Medium

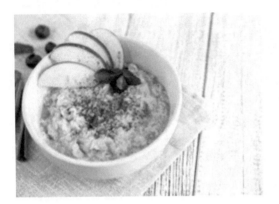

### Ingredients:

- ½ cup rolled oats
- ½ cup spring water
- ½ cup almond milk or any plant-based milk of your choice
- 1 tsp raw honey
- Pinch of cinnamon powder
- ½ small fuji apple, Peeled and sliced
- 5g almonds, chopped
- 5g walnuts, chopped

### Instructions:

1. Add rolled oats, water, and almond milk to a saucepan and cook for 7-10 minutes.
2. Serve in a bowl and add sliced apple and chopped nuts over it.
3. Serve immediately.

Total calories: 350 | Carbohydrates: 62g | Proteins: 10g | Fats: 15g

## 6. Healthy Avocado Toast

Prep Time: 7 min l Cook Time: 0 mins l Total Time: 15-20 mins l Difficulty: Easy

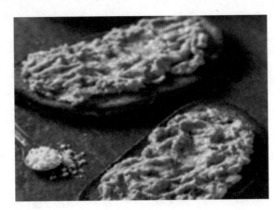

### Ingredients:

- One ripe avocado, pitted
- 1 tbsp extra virgin olive oil
- ¼ tsp turmeric powder
- Pinch of red chili flakes
- 1 tsp lemon juice
- ¼ cup cherry tomatoes, diced
- one slice of whole-grain bread
- Salt and pepper to taste

### Instructions:

1. First, toast the bread slice until it gets a golden-brown color.
2. Cut the avocado in half, scoop the flesh out of it, and mash it with a fork.
3. Add extra virgin olive oil, turmeric powder, salt, pepper, and lemon juice in the mashed avocado.
4. Spread the avocado mixture on the toast. Sprinkle a pinch of chili flakes. Top with cherry tomatoes.
5. Serve immediately.

Total calories: 570 | Carbohydrates: 38g | Proteins: 8g | Fats:46g

## 7. Hard Boiled eggs with Turmeric Milk

Prep Time: 7-10 min l Cook Time: 2-3 mins l Total Time: 15-20 mins l Difficulty: Easy

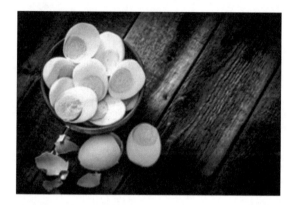

### Ingredients:

- One large egg
- For turmeric milk:
- 1 cup low-fat milk
- 1/8 tsp turmeric powder
- 1/8 tsp cinnamon powder
- 1 tsp raw honeyturmetic sauce

### Instructions:

Place egg in a saucepan with 2 cups of water on medium heat.
Let it cook for 10-12 minutes.
Place them in cold water. Peel off the shell and serve immediately.
Turmeric milk:
1. Boil 1 cup of milk with turmeric powder and cinnamon powder. Boil for 5-7 minutes.
2. Strain in a serving cup and serve while hot.
3. Serve immediately.

Total calories: 201 | Carbohydrates: 19g | Proteins: 15g | Fats: 8g

## 8. Walnut and flax seed energy-rich balls

Prep Time: 10-15 min l Cook Time: 0 mins l Total Time: 15-20 mins l Difficulty: easy

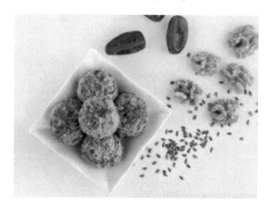

### Ingredients:

- ½ cup walnuts, crushed
- 1/8 cup rolled oats, ground in powder form
- 1 tbsp flax seeds
- 2 tbsp Peanut butter
- 1 tsp raw honey
- 3 Medjool dates, pitted
- 1/8 cup dried cranberries

### Instructions:

1. Mix all the ingredients in a bowl until well combined.
2. Shape them in the form of balls and roll them with the help of hands.
3. Serve immediately.

Total calories: 707 | Carbohydrates: 59g | Proteins: 18g | Fats:51g

# 9. White choc blueberry baked oatmeal

Prep Time: 10 min l Cook Time: 20 mins l Total Time: 30 mins l Difficulty: Easy

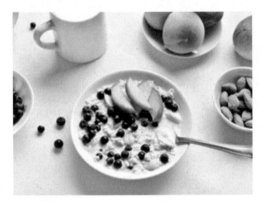

**Ingredients:**

- 1/2 banana
- 40g oats
- One whole egg
- 1/4 cup almond milk (or any other type of milk)
- 1 tbsp honey
- 1 tsp baking powder
- Some blueberries, peach and white choc chips for garnishing.

**Instructions:**

1. Preheat the oven to 180°C (356°F).
2. Mix all ingredients and bake in the oven for 20 minutes or until it turns golden brown.
3. Allow to cool lightly and serve!

Total calories: 296 | Carbohydrates: 37g | Proteins: 14g | Fats: 9g

# 10. Eggs in Purgatory

Prep Time: 10 min l Cook Time: 20-25 mins l Total Time: 30-35 mins l Difficulty: Medium

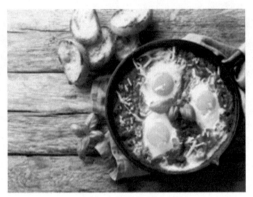

**Ingredients:**

- Canned tinned tomatoes - 1 can
- Onion 1 chopped
- Garlic 2 crushed
- Oregano 1 teaspoon
- Salt and pepper to taste
- Eggs 4

**Instructions:**

Turn the oven on to a temperature of 375°F.
In a large pan, heat the chopped onion and crushed garlic in some oil over medium heat until translucent and aromatic.
Pour the crushed tomatoes into the pan and add dried oregano, salt, and pepper. Cook for 5 to 7 minutes over low heat.
Now, make two dents in the basin of the tomato and break open two eggs in every dent.
Once completed, put the pot back in the hot oven so that the egg bakes for 20-25 minutes or until the egg is baked or firm.
When everything is done, take it out from the oven and allow it to rest for a bit before serving.

Total calories: 207 | Carbohydrates: 17g | Proteins: 15g | Fats:11g

# 1. Butternut Squash and Quinoa Soup

Prep Time: 15 minutes| Cook Time: 55 mins| Total Time: 1 hour 10 mins| Difficulty: Moderate

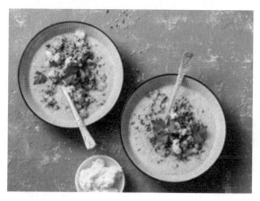

## Ingredients:
- ¼ small peeled and diced butternut squash
- ¼ cup quinoa
- ¼ onion (cut into small fragments)
- 2/3 tsp ginger garlic paste
- ¼ tsp turmeric
- 1 cup vegetable/chicken broth
- ½ tsp salt
- ¼ tsp black pepper
- Olive oil for cooking

## Instructions:
1. Preheat your oven to 400 degrees Fahrenheit.
2. Brush the diced butternut squash with olive oil and place it on a baking tray. Bake for 30 minutes or until tender.
3. Heat olive oil in a large pot and sauté the onion. As the onion starts to change color, add the ginger-garlic paste and turmeric. Cook for 2-3 minutes.
4. Then add rinsed quinoa with vegetable broth and let it boil. Simmer for 15-20 minutes so the quinoa cooks perfectly. Then add baked butternut squash. Heat again.
5. Season with salt and pepper. Serve hot and enjoy!

Total calories: 145 | Carbohydrates: 21g | Proteins: 4g | Fats: 6g

# 2. Tuscan Lentil Soup

Prep Time: 5 minutes| Cook Time: 25 mins| Total Time: 35 mins| Difficulty: Easy

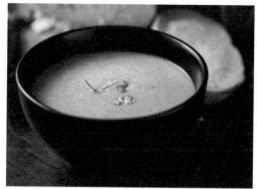

## Ingredients:
- ¼ cup lentils (dried)
- 1/3 can diced tomatoes
- ½ tsp basil
- ½ tsp oregano
- ¼ cup chopped spinach
- 1 cup vegetable broth
- 1 tsp ginger-garlic paste
- 1/3 tsp paprika
- ½ tsp salt
- ¼ tsp black pepper
- Olive oil for cooking

## Instructions:
1. Add olive oil into a pot and sauté onion. Then add ginger-garlic paste and sauté again until it softens.
2. Add tomatoes and basil and cook until they soften and break down, releasing their flavors. Then add oregano and paprika. Mix well.
3. Add rinsed lentils with vegetable broth and mix well to combine. Let the mixture boil, followed by simmering the mixture for 15-20 minutes until the lentils get soft.
4. Add salt and black pepper according to taste, and garnish with fresh basil.
5. Serve hot and enjoy!

Total calories: 240 | Carbohydrates: 31g | Proteins: 15g | Fats: 4g

## 3. Herbed Fisherman's Stew

Prep Time: 10 minutes| Cook Time: 22 mins| Total Time: 35 mins| Difficulty: Moderate

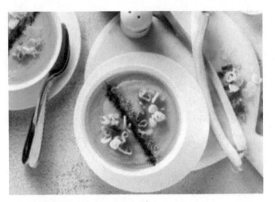

**Ingredients:**

- one small fennel bulb
- ½ tsp fennel seeds
- ½ chopped red onion
- 1 tsp ginger-garlic paste
- ½ tsp turmeric
- one small salmon fillet cut into chunks
- ¼ cup coconut milk
- 1.5 tsp olive oil
- 1 cup fish broth
- 1 tsp lemon juice
- Salt & pepper

**Instructions:**

1. Add olive oil to a pot and sauté onion. Then add sliced fennel bulbs, seeds, ginger-garlic paste, and sauté until softened.

2. Then add fish broth. Let it first boil and then simmer for 10 minutes.

3. Add salmon cubes to the pot and cook for 5 minutes or until the fish cubes are cooked.

4. Add coconut milk and half a lemon juice into the mixture and stir well. Cook for another 2 minutes to give a creamy touch.

5. Add salt and black pepper according to taste, and garnish with fresh dill.

6. Serve hot and enjoy!

Total calories: 610 | Carbohydrates: 11g | Proteins: 4.5g | Fats: 43g

## 4. Mediterranean Chickpea & Spinach Stew

Prep Time: 10 minutes| Cook Time: 12 mins| Total Time: 22 mins| Difficulty: Easy

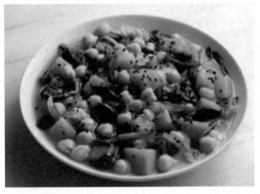

**Ingredients:**

- 1/2 cup chickpeas, rinsed
- 1/2 cup fresh spinach leaves
- 1/4 cup diced red bell pepper
- 1/4 cup Kalamata olives, pitted
- 2 garlic cloves, minced
- 1 tablespoon of olive oil
- 1 teaspoon of lemon juice
- 1/2 teaspoon ground cumin
- Salt and pepper to taste
- 1/4 teaspoon cayenne pepper

**Instructions:**

1. Take a pot and add olive oil to it. Put the pot over medium heat.

2. Add the garlic, cumin, and cayenne pepper. Cook for 1-2 minutes.

3. Then add the chickpeas, red bell pepper, and cucumber. Cook for 2-3 minutes.

4. Incorporate the spinach leaves into the pot and keep cooking.

5. Once the spinach leaves are wilted, stir in the lemon juice and mix well.

6. Season with salt and pepper to taste.

7. Garnish with Kalamata olives and serve immediately to enjoy the stew while it's still hot.

Total calories: 305 | Carbohydrates: 33g | Proteins: 11g | Fats: 16g

## 5. Turmeric-infused chicken and Yam Gratin

Prep Time: 10 minutes| Cook Time: 22 mins| Total Time: 35 mins| Difficulty: Moderate

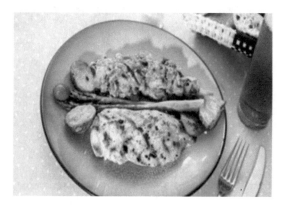

**Ingredients:**

- 1 small chicken breast (boneless)
- 1 medium sweet potato, peeled and diced
- 1 tablespoon of olive oil
- 1 teaspoon of ground turmeric
- 1/2 teaspoon ground ginger
- 1/4 teaspoon black pepper
- ¼ tsp cayenne pepper
- ¼ teaspoon Boswellia resin, optional
- 1/4 cup chopped fresh cilantro

**Instructions:**

1. Preheat the oven to 400 degrees Fahrenheit.
2. In a large bowl, toss the chicken and sweet potato with olive oil, turmeric, ginger, black pepper, Boswellia resin, and cayenne pepper.
3. Line a baking sheet with parchment paper. Add the mixture to the sheet and spread evenly.
4. Roast in the oven for 25-30 minutes or until you ensure your chicken and sweet potato are adequately cooked and tender.
5. Take the baked chicken and sweet potato out of the oven and garnish with cilantro.
6. Serve hot and enjoy!

Total calories: 433 | Carbohydrates: 26g | Proteins: 40g | Fats: 17g

## 6. Creamy Avocado Pesto Pasta

Prep Time: 15 minutes| Cook Time: 20 mins| Total Time: 35 mins| Difficulty: Moderate

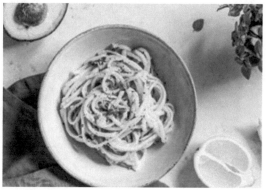

**Ingredients:**

- 2 oz (about 1/4 cup) whole wheat or gluten-free pasta of your choice
- 1/2 ripe avocado
- 1/4 cup fresh basil leaves
- one small garlic clove
- 1 tbsp lemon juice
- 1 tbsp nutritional yeast
- 1 tbsp olive oil
- 1/2 tsp turmeric powder
- 1 tbsp pine nuts or walnuts
- 1/2 cup baby spinach or arugula
- Cherry tomatoes, halved

**Instructions:**

1. Take a pot and add olive oil to it. Put the pot over medium heat.
2. Add the garlic, cumin, and cayenne pepper. Cook for 1-2 minutes.
3. Then add the chickpeas, red bell pepper, and cucumber. Cook for 2-3 minutes.
4. Incorporate the spinach leaves into the pot and keep cooking.
5. Once the spinach leaves are wilted, stir in the lemon juice and mix well.
6. Season with salt and pepper to taste.
7. Garnish with Kalamata olives.

Total calories: 305 | Carbohydrates: 33g | Proteins: 11g | Fats: 16g

## 7. Anti-Inflammatory Brown Rice Bowl

Prep Time: 10 minutes|Cook Time: 20 mins| Total Time: 30 mins| Difficulty: Easy

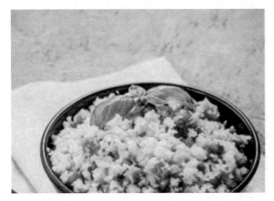

**Ingredients:**

- 1/2 cup cooked brown rice
- 1/2 cup cauliflower florets
- 1/4 tsp turmeric powder
- 1/4 tsp ground cumin
- 1 tbsp olive oil
- one small carrot, sliced
- 1/4 cup chickpeas
- 1 tbsp pumpkin seeds or sunflower seeds
- Salt and pepper to taste
- 1 tbsp tahini sauce
- 1 tsp lemon juice
- 1 tsp water

**Instructions:**

1. Coat the cauliflower florets with olive oil, turmeric, and other seasonings. Arrange them on the baking sheet and put them in the preheated oven.
2. Place the cooked brown rice in a serving bowl as the base. Arrange the roasted cauliflower, sliced carrot, and chickpeas on top.
3. Whisk the tahini, lemon juice, water, salt, and pepper. Add water to adjust the thickness.
4. Drizzle the tahini dressing over the bowl. Finally, add pumpkin seeds for a crunchier texture.
5. Garnish with fresh parsley and serve.

Total Calories: 433 Carbohydrates: 46g Proteins: 11g Fat: 25g

## 8. Quinoa Royale

Prep Time: 10 minutes|Cook Time: 20 mins| Total Time: 30 mins| Difficulty: Easy

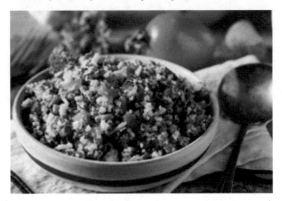

**Ingredients:**

- ¼ cup quinoa, rinsed and drained
- ½ cup of anti-inflammatory herbal tea
- ½ tbsp olive oil
- ¼ small red onion, finely chopped
- one small garlic clove, minced
- ¼ tsp turmeric powder
- ¼ tsp ground cumin
- ¼ cup zucchini, diced
- ¼ cup bell pepper, diced
- Salt and pepper to taste
- 1 tbsp fresh parsley or cilantro

**Instructions:**

1. Rinse the quinoa and cook it using the herbal tea according to the instructions given on the package.
2. Add olive oil to a pot and heat it over medium flame. Add and sauté the red onions and garlic for 2-3 minutes. Next, add the spices, turmeric, and cumin, stirring for another minute.
3. Add veggies and cook for 5-7 minutes. The veggies will get tender but slightly crisp.
4. Add the cooked quinoa to the pot, stirring well to combine—season with salt and pepper to taste.
5. Transfer the quinoa pilaf to a serving bowl and top with fresh parsley. Serve and enjoy.

Total Calories: 145 Carbs: 15g Proteins: 3g Fat: 8g

# 1. Thai Pumpkin Broth

Prep Time: 15 minutes|Cook Time: 4 hrs.| Total Time: 4 | Difficulty: Easy

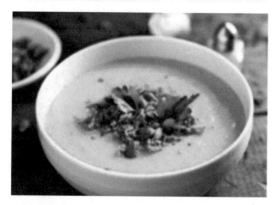

## Ingredients:

- 1/2 cup pumpkin puree
- 1/2 cup coconut milk
- 1/4 cup vegetable broth
- 1/2 tbsp olive oil
- two tablespoons of Thai red curry paste
- 1/2 teaspoon ground cumin
- 1/2 teaspoon turmeric powder
- Salt and pepper to taste
- Fresh cilantro leaves for garnish

## Instructions:

1. Place all the ingredients in your slow cooker.
2. Set the cooker to low heat and cook for 3-4 hours.
3. Taste and adjust seasoning as needed.
4. Serve hot, garnished with fresh cilantro leaves.

Total Calories: 132 Carbohydrates: 16g
Proteins: 3g  Fat: 8g

# 2. Classic Lamb Roast

Prep Time: 12 minutes|Cook Time: 6 hrs| Total Time 6 hrs 12 min| Difficulty: Easy

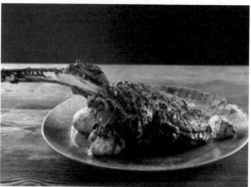

## Ingredients:

- 4 lb boneless lamb meat (shoulder/leg meat with excess fat removed)
- 1/2 tbsp olive oil
- 1 tsp turmeric powder
- 1 tsp ginger powder
- 1 tsp cinnamon powder
- 1/2 tsp black pepper
- 1/4 cup chopped fresh rosemary
- two cloves garlic, minced
- 1/4 tsp dried thyme
- 1/4 tsp sea salt
- 1/4 cup pomegranate juice
- 1 tbsp apple cider vinegar
- 1 tbsp fresh mint

## Instructions:

1. Season the lamb with salt, turmeric, ginger, cinnamon, and black pepper.
2. Warm the olive oil in a skillet set to medium-high heat. Cook the lamb until it is browned evenly on each side, roughly 2-3 minutes per side.
3. Transfer the lamb to the slow cooker. Add rosemary and garlic and mix well. Then, add liquids, such as apple cider vinegar and pomegranate juice.
4. Cover and cook on low for 6-8 hours or until the lamb is tender and easily shredded with a fork.
5. Serve hot and enjoy.

Total Calories: 385 Carbohydrates: 13g
Proteins: 3g  Fat: 29g

## 3. Savory Vegetable Casserole

Prep Time: 15 minutes|Cook Time: 4 hrs| Total Time: 4 hr 15 mins| Difficulty: Easy

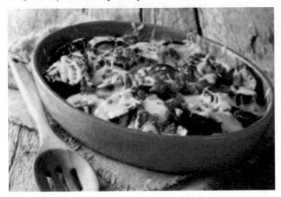

**Ingredients:**

- 1/4 small eggplant, diced
- 1/4 small zucchini, sliced into rounds
- 1/4 red bell pepper, diced
- 1/4 yellow bell pepper, diced
- 1/4 small red onion, sliced
- one small tomato, diced
- one small garlic clove, minced
- 1 tbsp olive oil
- 1/4 tsp dried thyme
- 1/4 tsp smoked paprika
- 1/4 cup low-sodium vegetable broth
- 1 tbsp balsamic vinegar
- 1 tsp honey

**Instructions:**

1. In a small bowl, mix the diced vegetables with olive oil, minced garlic, thyme, turmeric, paprika, and lemon juice and toss to coat.

2. Add these marinated veggies to a slow cooker.

3. Combine broth, balsamic vinegar, and honey to make a saucy liquid. Pour it evenly over the veggies in the cooker.

4. Cover the cooker for 4-5 hours until the vegetables are cooked properly and all the flavors are released and combined.

5. Once cooked, give the ratatouille a gentle stir. Serve hot, garnished with lemon wedges.

Total Calories: 213 Carbohydrates: 23g Proteins: 2g  Fat: 14g

## 4. Oats and Berry Bowl

Prep Time: 15 minutes|Cook Time: 4-5 hrs| Total Time: 4 hr 15 mins| Difficulty: Easy

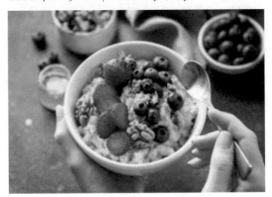

**Ingredients:**

- For Oatmeal:
- 1/4 cup steel-cut oats
- 1 cup almond milk (unsweetened)
- 1/2 tsp ground turmeric (anti-inflammatory boost)
- 1/4 tsp ground cinnamon
- 1/2 tsp vanilla extract
- 1 tbsp honey
- For Toppings:
- 1/4 cup mixed berries
- 1 tbsp chopped walnuts or almonds
- 1 tsp chia seeds
- 1 tbsp coconut flakes

**Instructions:**

1. Combine all the oatmeal ingredients in a cooker and mix well.

2. Cover the cooker and cook for 4-5 hours. For a creamier texture, you can incorporate additional almond milk while cooking.

3. In a bowl, top the cooked oatmeal with mixed berries, walnuts, chia seeds, and coconut flakes.

4. Serve and enjoy your warm, anti-inflammatory oatmeal as a nourishing breakfast.

Total Calories: 312 Carbohydrates: 40g  Proteins: 9g  Fat: 13

## 5. Cozy Sweet Potato Chili

Prep Time: 15 minutes|Cook Time: 4 hrs| Total Time: 4 hrs 15 mins| Difficulty: Moderate

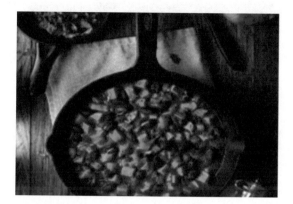

### Ingredients:

* one small, sweet potato, peeled and diced
* 1/4 cup cooked black beans
* 1/4 cup diced tomatoes
* 1/4 cup vegetable broth
* 1/4 teaspoon turmeric
* 1/4 teaspoon cumin
* 1/4 teaspoon paprika
* Salt and pepper to taste
* Fresh cilantro for garnish

### Instructions:

1. Place the diced sweet potato, black beans, tomatoes, and vegetable broth in the slow cooker.
2. Add the turmeric, cumin, paprika, salt, and pepper. Stir to combine.
3. Cook on low heat for 4-6 hours or until the sweet potatoes are tender.
4. After cooking, taste the dish and adjust the seasonings as necessary.
5. Serve the chili hot, garnished with fresh cilantro.

Total Calories: 125 Carbohydrates: 25g
Proteins: 6g Fat: 0g

## 6. Anti-inflammatory Meatballs

Prep Time: 15 minutes| Cook Time: 4 hrs | Total Time: 4 hrs 15 mins| Difficulty: Moderate

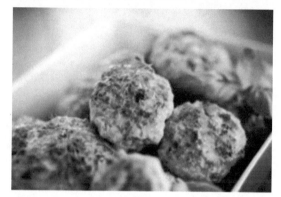

### Ingredients:

* ¼ pound ground chicken (lean meat)
* ¼ cup finely chopped onion
* one clove of garlic, minced
* ½ teaspoon turmeric
* ½ teaspoon ground ginger
* ¼ teaspoon black pepper
* ¼ teaspoon dried oregano
* ¼ teaspoon dried basil
* ¼ cup low-sodium chicken broth
* ¼ cup chopped tomatoes

### Instructions:

1. Mix the ground turkey or chicken with the chopped onion, minced garlic, turmeric, ginger, black pepper, oregano, and basil until well combined.
2. Form the mixture into meatballs of the desired size.
3. Place the meatballs in the slow cooker.
4. Pour the low-sodium chicken broth and chopped tomatoes over the meatballs.
5. Cook on low for 4-6 hours until the meatballs are edible & cooked.
6. Serve the anti-inflammatory meatballs hot and enjoy!

Total calories: 265 Carbohydrates: 11gProteins: 28g Fat: 13g

## 7. Coconut Vegetable Curry

Prep Time: 15 minutes|Cook Time: 2 hrs| Total Time: 2 hrs 15 mins| Difficulty: Moderate

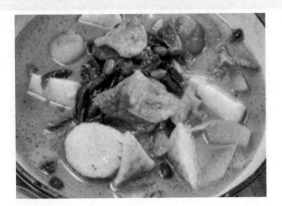

### Ingredients:

- ½ cup mixed vegetables (e.g., colorful bell peppers, carrots, and zucchini)
- ¼ cup coconut milk
- ½ teaspoon turmeric
- ½ teaspoon ground ginger
- ¼ teaspoon cumin
- ¼ teaspoon coriander
- ¼ teaspoon paprika
- Salt and pepper to taste

### Instructions:

1. Add all the ingredients except vegetables in a bowl. Mix well to make a coconut milk mixture.
2. Then, keep the mixed veggies in a slow cooker. Add and drizzle the coconut milk mixture over the veggies, mixing well to ensure the veggies are well combined with the mixture.
3. Cover the cooker and let the veggies cook for 2-3 hours or until they're tender and edible.
4. Take out the curry into a bowl and serve hot.

Total calories: 145 Carbohydrates: 9g Proteins: 3g   Fat: 13g

## 8. Nutmeggie Lasagna

Prep Time: 15 minutes|Cook Time: 4 hrs| Total Time: 4 hrs 15 mins| Difficulty: Moderate

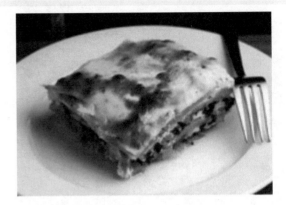

### Ingredients:

- two whole-wheat lasagna noodles
- ¼ cup low-fat ricotta cheese
- ¼ cup marinara sauce
- ¼ cup diced vegetables (such as zucchini, bell peppers, and spinach)
- ¼ teaspoon dried oregano
- ¼ teaspoon dried basil
- ¼ tsp nutmeg
- 1 tsp balsamic vinegar
- Salt and pepper to taste

### Instructions:

1. Add ricotta cheese to a bowl and mix it with oregano, basil, nutmeg, and balsamic vinegar. Then, add salt and pepper to the bowl as needed. Combine well to create a flavorful ricotta mixture.
2. Next, take a cooker and start layering it. The first layer is marinara sauce, then add the lasagna noodles layer, followed by the ricotta mixture you prepared. Finally, the last layer is of veggies. Keep repeating the layering process until the ingredients are finished.
3. Start heating the cooker slowly for 3-4 hours. Turn off the flame once the noodles are tender and veggies are cooked.
4. Serve hot, and enjoy.

Total calories: 295   Carbohydrates: 48g  Proteins: 14g Fat: 4g

# 1. Black Bean Zucchini and Corn Salad

Prep Time: 15 minutes|Cook Time: 2 mins| Total Time: 17 mins| Difficulty: Easy

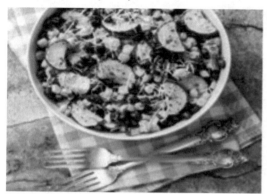

## Ingredients:

- ½ cup canned black beans
- One medium zucchini diced
- ½ cup corn, fresh or frozen as per choice
- 1/8 cup fresh cilantro leaves
- ¼ cup parmesan cheese (for topping)
- For Dressing:
- 1 tbsp avocado oil
- one teaspoon of lime juice
- Sea salt and black pepper as per taste
- one clove of garlic, minced
- ¼ tsp cumin powder

## Instructions:

1.Stir-fry sliced zucchini in a pan with 1 tsp of extra virgin olive oil for 1-2 minutes.
2.Combine black beans, zucchini, corn, and fresh cilantro leaves in a bowl.
3.Add salad dressing over it. Mix well.
4.Serve immediately.

Total calories: 444 Carbohydrates: 45g
Proteins: 20g  Fat: 23g

# 2. Whole wheat broccoli spaghetti salad with Herbed Salmon

Prep Time: 15 minutes|Cook Time: 20 mins| Total Time: 35 mins| Difficulty: Moderate

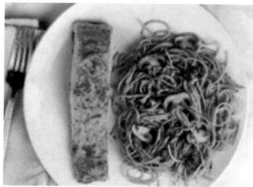

## Ingredients:

- For the spaghetti
- 60g whole wheat spaghetti, boiled
- ½ cup broccoli florets
- ¼ cup cherry tomatoes, diced
- ¼ cup mushrooms
- 1 tsp extra virgin olive oil
- For the salmon:
- One salmon fillet (6oz, 170g)
- 1 tsp extra virgin olive oil
- ¼ tsp garlic powder
- ¼ tsp dried thyme
- ½ tsp dried dill

## Instructions:

1.Marinate the salmon fillet with the mentioned ingredients and leave it for 20 minutes.
2.Grease the pan with extra virgin olive oil and cook the salmon fillet on medium heat for 5 minutes on each side or until thoroughly cooked.
3. Boil the whole wheat spaghetti according to the package instructions. Add the boiled spaghetti, broccoli florets, and cherry tomatoes to a bowl. Drizzle apple cider vinegar, dried oregano, and freshly ground black pepper over it and mix it well. Serve hot and enjoy!

Total calories: 566 Carbohydrates: 27g
Proteins: 44g Fat: 31g

## 3. Raw Beet & Arugula Salad with Walnuts

Prep Time: 15 minutes|Cook Time: 0 mins| Total Time: 15 mins| Difficulty: Easy

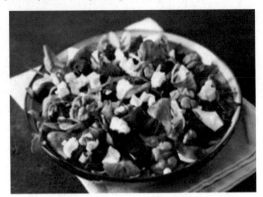

### Ingredients:

- One small beetroot, peeled and chopped
- One cup radicchio, chopped
- ½ cup arugula
- 5g chopped walnuts
- 1 tsp extra virgin olive oil
- 1 tsp apple cider vinegar
- Few cilantro leaves
- Freshly ground black pepper as per taste
- ¼ cup feta cheese
- 1 tsp lime juice

### Instructions:

1. Combine the salad ingredients in a bowl.
2. Combine lime juice, apple cider vinegar, black pepper, and olive oil and drizzle over the salad.
3. Top it with cilantro, walnuts, and feta cheese. Serve immediately.

Total calories: 206  Carbohydrates: 9g Proteins: 8g Fat: 16g

## 4. Turmeric Cauliflower & Quinoa Salad

Prep Time: 15 minutes|Cook Time: 20 mins| Total Time: 35 mins| Difficulty: Moderate

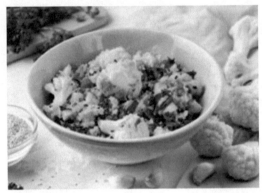

### Ingredients:

- ½ cup quinoa, rinsed
- ½ cup cauliflower florets
- one small red onion, chopped
- ¼ cup cilantro leaves
- ¼ cup cherry tomatoes
- Pinch of turmeric powder
- ¼ tsp cumin powder
- For the dressing:
- 1 tbsp tahini
- 1 tsp lime juice
- 1 tsp balsamic vinegar
- 1/4 tsp black pepper
- 1 tsp extra virgin olive oil

### Instructions:

1. Cook the quinoa. Add the rinsed quinoa and spring water to a pan and boil on medium heat.
2. Let it cook for about 15-20 minutes. Set it aside.
3. Stir-fry cauliflower florets in a small pan with turmeric and cumin powder for 2 minutes. Add cooked quinoa, stir-fry cauliflower, red onion, and diced cherry tomatoes in a bowl.
Season with turmeric and cumin
4. Drizzle dressing over the salad. Mix evenly, and serve immediately.

Total calories: 290  Carbohydrates: 34g Proteins: 9g  Fat: 15g

## 5. Mixed Berry Spinach Salad with walnuts

Prep Time: 10 minutes|Cook Time: 0 mins| Total Time: 10 mins| Difficulty: Easy

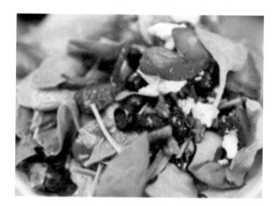

### Ingredients:

- 1 cup baby spinach leaves
- ½ cup strawberries, halved
- ½ cup blueberries
- 5g walnuts
- Pinch of cinnamon powder
- ¼ cup feta cheese
- 1 tsp acacia honey

### Instructions:

1. Combine all the ingredients in a bowl.
2. Top it with walnuts, cinnamon powder, and feta cheese.
3. Serve immediately.

## 6. Basil broccoli pasta salad

Prep Time: 15 minutes|Cook Time: 10 mins| Total Time: 25 mins| Difficulty: Moderate

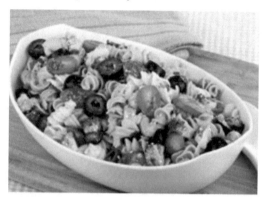

### Ingredients:

- 1 cup whole wheat pasta, boiled
- ½ cup broccoli florets
- ¼ cup cherry tomatoes
- 2 tbsp black olives
- ½ small cucumber, diced
- For the dressing:
- 2 tbsp low-fat mayonnaise
- 4 tbsp yogurt
- ¼ tsp black pepper
- ¼ tsp sea salt
- 1 tsp extra virgin olive oil
- ½ tsp basil leaves

### Instructions:

1. Boil the pasta as per package instructions.
1. Combine all the ingredients in a bowl.
2. Drizzle the dressing over the salad.
3. Serve immediately.

Total calories: 230 Carbohydrates: 26g Proteins: 8g Fat: 12g

Total calories: 394 Carbohydrates: 54g Proteins: 13g Fat: 16g

## 7. Kohlrabi, Cucumber & Carrot Coleslaw

Prep Time: 15 minutes|Cook Time: 0 mins| Total Time: 15 mins| Difficulty: Easy

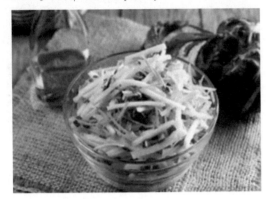

**Ingredients:**

- one small kohlrabi peeled and (cut in julienned form)
- one small cucumber peeled and (cut in julienned form)
- one medium carrot peeled and (cut in julienned form)
- one small green apple peeled and (cut in julienned form)
- 1 tsp lime juice
- 1/8 tsp sea salt
- ¼ tsp black pepper
- 1 tsp fresh parsley, chopped

**Instructions:**

1. Combine all the ingredients in a bowl.
2. Add lime juice, sea salt, black pepper, and fresh parsley over the salad.
3. Serve immediately.

## 8. Raw kale with edamame beans and carrot salad

Prep Time: 10 minutes|Cook Time: 0 mins| Total Time: 10 mins| Difficulty: Easy

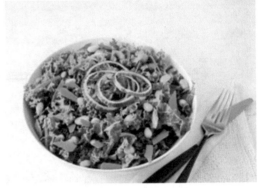

**Ingredients:**

- 1 cup raw kale, chopped
- ½ cup shelled edamame beans, cooked
- one medium carrot, peeled and grated
- For the dressing:
- 1 tbsp lime juice
- 1 tsp extra virgin olive oil
- ¼ tsp black pepper
- 1/8 tsp cayenne pepper

**Instructions:**

1. Combine all the ingredients in a bowl.
2. Add lime juice, extra virgin olive oil, black pepper, and cayenne pepper over the salad.
3. Serve immediately.

Total calories: 161  Carbohydrates: 40g  Proteins: 4g  Fat: 1g

Total calories: 190  Carbohydrates: 19g  Proteins: 12g  Fat: 9g

# CHAPTER 3

## *FAMILY-FRIENDLY MEALS*

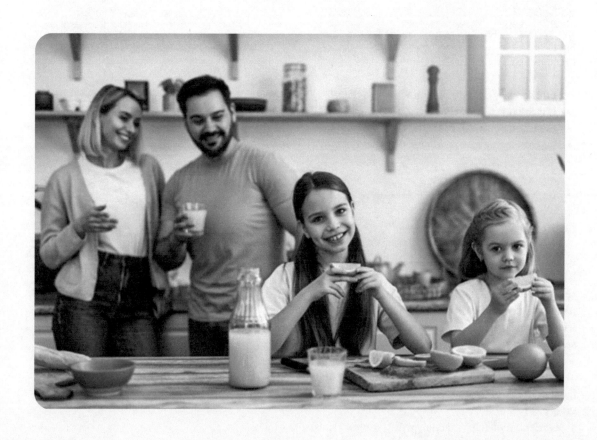

# 1. Smoked Paprika Sweet potato fries

Prep Time: 10 minutes|Cook Time: 20 mins| Total Time: 30 mins| Difficulty: Easy

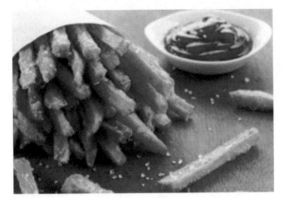

## Ingredients:

- 1 medium-sized sweet potato
- 1 teaspoon extra virgin olive oil
- 1 teaspoon corn-starch
- 1/4 teaspoon garlic powder
- Sea Salt as per taste
- Black pepper as per taste
- 1/2 teaspoon smoked paprika powder

## Instructions:

1. Peel the sweet potato and cut into the shape of thin fries or wedges as per your choice.
2. Preheat your oven to 220 C and place parchment paper on the baking sheet. In a bowl, add sweet potato fries, extra virgin olive oil, cornstarch, garlic powder, sea salt, black pepper, and smoked paprika. Toss them well.
3. Place the seasoned fries on the baking sheet and bake in the oven for 20-25 minutes until they get crispy.
5. Serve immediately and enjoy with a dipping sauce of your favorite choice.

Total calories: 161   Carbohydrates: 27g   Proteins: 3g   Fat: 5g

# 2. Kiwi & Mango Greek Yogurt Parfait

Prep Time: 15 minutes|Cook Time: 0 mins| Total Time: 15 mins| Difficulty: Easy

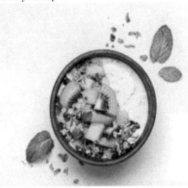

## Ingredients:

- ½ cup low-fat or plain Greek yogurt
- One small kiwi, peeled and sliced
- ½ Fresh mango, peeled and cubed
- ¼ cup granola
- 5g almonds, crushed
- 5g walnuts, crushed
- 1 tbsp manuka honey (Optional)

## Instructions:

1. Add ¼ cup Greek yogurt in a bowl, then layer kiwi, mango chunks, and granola.
2. Repeat the same layer.
3. Top it with crushed almonds & walnuts on top.
4. Refrigerate in the fridge for 30 minutes & enjoy.

Total calories: 434  Carbohydrates: 61g   Proteins: 19g   Fat: 15g

## 3. Mango and blueberry smoothie bowl with mixed nuts

Prep Time: 10 minutes|Cook Time: 20 mins| Total Time: 30 mins| Difficulty: Easy

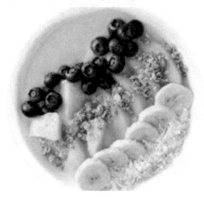

### Ingredients:

- ½ cup fresh or frozen mango chunks
- ¼ cup blueberries
- ½ small banana, sliced
- ½ cup almond milk or any plant-based milk of your choice
- 2 tbsp. rolled oats
- 5g pecans
- 1 tbsp shredded coconut
- 1 tsp basil seeds (soaked in water for 15-20 minutes)
- Ice cubes as needed

### Instructions:

1. Place all ingredients except chia seeds in a blender.
2. Blend quickly until you achieve a smooth and creamy consistency.
3. Pour this smoothie mixture into a bowl. Top it with crushed pecans and soaked basil seeds.
4. Serve immediately.

Total calories: 262 Carbohydrates: 46g Proteins: 5g   Fat: 9g

## 4. Chicken Veggie Pita Pockets

Prep Time: 10 minutes|Cook Time: 5 mins| Total Time:15 mins| Difficulty: Easy

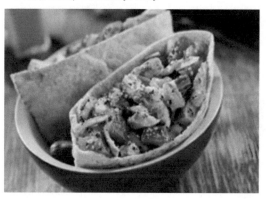

### Ingredients:

- One small whole-wheat pita bread
- ½ cup shredded chicken
- ¼ cup carrot, peeled and grated
- ¼ cup diced bell pepper
- ¼ cup shredded cabbage
- 2 tbsp olives (Green or black)
- 1 tsp extra virgin olive oil
- ¼ tsp turmeric powder
- ¼ tsp cumin powder
- Salt and black pepper as per taste

### Instructions:

1. Heat olive oil over medium heat in a small pan. Add cumin powder, black pepper, and salt. 2. Add the shredded chicken, grated carrots, bell pepper, olives, and cabbage in the pan and cook for 2-3 minutes.
3. cut the pita bread in half and add the chicken-vegetable mixture. Your chicken-vegetable pita pocket is ready to serve.

Total calories: 281 Carbohydrates: 25g Proteins: 21g Fat: 12g

## 5. Tropical Spinach Fusion Smoothie

Prep Time: 10 minutes|Cook Time: 0 mins| Total Time: 10 mins| Difficulty: Easy

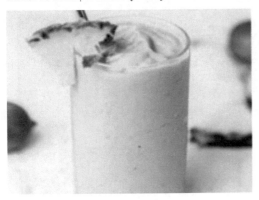

### Ingredients:

- 1 cup frozen baby spinach leaves
- ½ cup frozen pineapple chunks
- ¼ cup mango chunks
- ½ cup almond milk
- One tsp manuka honey
- Pinch of cinnamon powder
- 1 tsp hemp seeds
- 5g Brazil nuts

### Instructions:

1. Blend all the ingredients quickly until you achieve a smooth and creamy consistency.
2. If the smoothie is too thick, add half a cup of coconut water to adjust the consistency.
3. Serve immediately.

Total calories: 204  Carbohydrates: 36g  Proteins: 4g  Fat: 7g

## 6. Mixed Rainbow fruit skewers

Prep Time: 10 minutes|Cook Time: 0 mins| Total Time: 10 mins| Difficulty: Eas

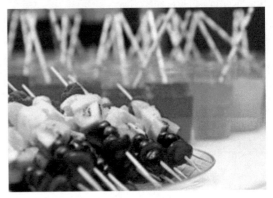

### Ingredients:

- one large strawberry halved
- four cherries, pitted
- one-two-inch piece of pineapple
- one-two-inch piece of cantaloupe
- two blueberries
- 2-3 grapes
- A one-inch piece of kiwi, peeled and sliced

### Instructions:

1. Take a wooden skewer and arrange the fruits individually, starting with halved strawberries, cherries, cubed pineapple and cantaloupe, grapes, blueberries, and kiwi.
2. Serve immediately.

Total calories: 101 Carbohydrates: 25g  Proteins: 2g  Fat: 0 g

## 7. Green Kiwi & Pear Smoothie

Prep Time: 8 minutes|Cook Time: 0 mins| Total Time: 8 mins| Difficulty: Easy

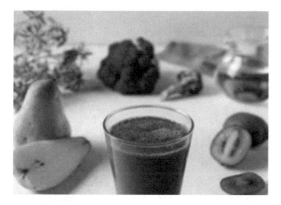

**Ingredients:**

- one small ripe kiwi
- one small pear, peeled & chopped
- one cup of sparkling water
- ¼ cup broccoli florets
- 1 tsp raw honey
- Pinch of turmeric powder
- One tsp chia seeds soaked in water for 5-10 minutes

**Instructions:**

1. Blend all the ingredients at high speed until you achieve your desired consistency.
3. Serve this smoothie in a glass and garnish it with a slice of kiwi.
3. Serve immediately.

## 8. Mixed berries and Peach skewers with dark chocolate drizzle

Prep Time: 8 minutes|Cook Time: 0 mins| Total Time: 8 mins| Difficulty: Easy

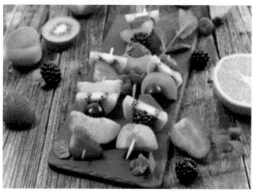

**Ingredients:**

- Two strawberries, halved
- Two raspberries
- Two blueberries
- Two blackberries
- One-inch piece of peach, cubed
- One-inch piece of mango, cubed
- 1 tsp dark chocolate syrup (for drizzle)

**Instructions:**

1. Take a wooden skewer and arrange the fruits individually, starting with halved strawberries, raspberries, blueberries, blackberries, peaches, and mango.
2. Drizzle chocolate syrup over it.
3. Serve immediately.

Total calories: 169 Carbohydrates: 40g
Proteins: 3g Fat: 2g

Total calories: 63  Carbohydrates: 15g
Proteins: 1g  Fat: 0g

## 1. Cherries & avocado mousse

Prep Time: 10 minutes|Chill Time: 60 mins| Total Time: 70 mins| Difficulty: Easy

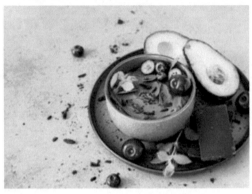

### Ingredients:

- ½ ripe avocado
- ½ cup frozen cherries, pitted
- Two tablespoons of cacao powder
- ¼ cup spring water
- 2 Medjool dates
- 5g walnuts
- One tsp acacia honey or maple syrup
- Pinch of cinnamon powder

### Instructions:

1. Combine all the ingredients in a high-speed blender and blend until smooth.
2. Pour the mixture into a serving jar or bowl and chill it for 30-60 min before serving.

## 2. Strawberry Creamed Cottage Cheese mousse

Prep Time: 10 minutes|Chill Time: 60 mins| Total Time: 70 mins| Difficulty: Easy

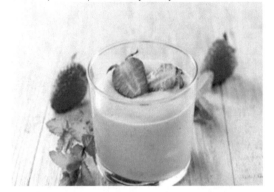

### Ingredients:

- ½ cup strawberries
- ½ cup of creamed cottage cheese
- 1 tbsp. Maple syrup or manuka honey
- Strawberries for topping
- ¼ cup almond milk

### Instructions:

1. Combine strawberries, almond milk, and honey in a blender. Blend well until it gets smooth.
2. Beat the creamed cottage cheese until it gets fluffy.
3. now mix both the mixtures and divide them into two serving jars or bowls. Refrigerate it for 1 hour before serving.
4. Top with fresh strawberry chunks on top

Total calories: 437  Carbohydrates: 67g Proteins 7g  Fat: 20g

Total calories: 213 Carbohydrates: 29g Proteins: 14g  Fat: 5g

## 3. Kiwi & Banana Greek Yogurt Parfait

Prep Time: 12 minutes|Cook Time: 0 mins| Total Time: 12 mins| Difficulty: Easy

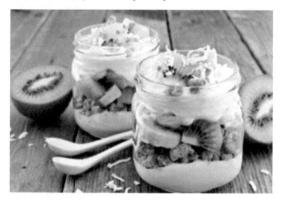

**Ingredients:**

- One small kiwi, peeled & sliced
- ½ banana, sliced
- ½ cup plain low-fat yogurt or Greek yogurt
- 2 tbsp. graham crackers
- 1 tbsp shredded coconut
- 5g walnuts, crushed

**Instructions:**

1. Add ¼ cup Greek yogurt in a bowl, then layer kiwi, sliced banana, and crushed graham crackers.
2. Repeat the same layer.
3. Top it with crushed walnuts & shredded coconut.
4. Refrigerate in the fridge for 30 minutes & enjoy.

Total calories: 337Carbohydrates: 52gProteins: 16g    Fat: 9g

## 4. Mango & Blackberry Greek Yogurt Parfait

Prep Time: 12 minutes|Cook Time: 0 mins| Total Time: 12 mins| Difficulty: Easy

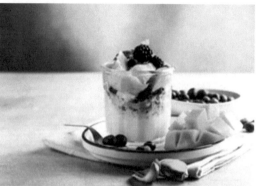

**Ingredients:**

- ¼ cup mango chunks
- ½ cup blackberries
- ½ cup plain low-fat yogurt or Greek yogurt
- 2 tbsp. granola
- 1 tsp chia seeds (soaked in water for 5-10 mins)
- 5g cashews (or any other nuts), crushed

**Instructions:**

1. Add ¼ cup Greek yogurt in a bowl, then layer mango, blackberries, and granola.
2. Repeat the same layer.
3. Top it with crushed cashews and chia seeds.
4. Refrigerate in the fridge for 30 minutes & enjoy.

Total calories: 241Carbohydrates: 28gProteins: 16g    Fat: 8g

## 5. Crunchy Peachy Yogurt Parfait

Prep Time: 12 minutes|Cook Time: 0 mins| Total Time: 12 mins| Difficulty: Easy

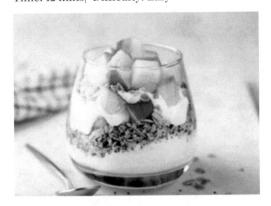

**Ingredients:**

- ½ cup Greek yogurt
- One small peach, cubed
- ¼ cup pineapple chunks
- 2 tbsp granola
- 5g crushed pecans
- 1 tsp flax seeds

**Instructions:**

1. Add ¼ cup Greek yogurt in a bowl, then layer half of the peach, pineapple chunks, and granola.
2. Repeat the same layer.
3. Top it with crushed pecans and flax seeds.
4. Refrigerate in the fridge for 30 minutes & enjoy.

.

total calories: 282  Carbohydrates: 36gProteins: 16g    Fat: 10g

## 6. Apple Cinnamon Pudding with Almonds Topping

Prep Time: 10 minutes|Cook Time: 0 mins| Total Time: 70 mins| Difficulty: Easy

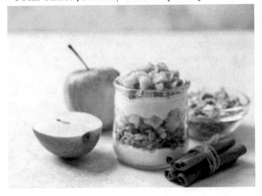

**Ingredients:**

- one small apple, diced
- ¼ cup almond milk
- 1 tbsp. manuka honey
- 1/8 tsp cinnamon powder
- 1 tbsp. granola
- 1 tbsp chia seeds

**Instructions:**

1. Mix all the ingredients well in a bowl and leave it in a refrigerator for 2 hours.
2. Top it with granola and fresh apple chunks.

Total calories: 258  Carbohydrates: 49gProteins: 4g  Fat: 6g

## 7. Zucchini & Beet Brownies

Prep Time: 10 minutes|Cook Time: 20 mins| Total Time: 30 mins| Difficulty: Easy

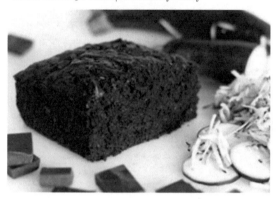

### Ingredients:

- ½ small zucchini, peeled and grated
- ½ small beetroot, peeled and grated
- ¼ cup whole wheat flour
- 2 tbsp. cocoa powder
- ¼ cup almond butter
- one medium egg
- ¼ tsp baking powder
- 1 tsp maple syrup
- ¼ tsp vanilla extract
- 2 tbsp dark chocolate chips
- 5g walnuts

### Instructions:

1. In a bowl, combine grated zucchini, beets, almond butter, egg, and maple syrup. Mix the remaining ingredients until the batter is well combined. Fold in dark chocolate chips and crushed walnuts.
2. Preheat oven to 175 C. Grease the baking dish with 1 tsp extra virgin olive oil.
3. Place the batter in the prepared baking dish and bake for 20-25 mins.
4. Serve immediately.

Total calories: 778 Carbohydrates: 62gProteins: 28g Fat: 51g

## 8. Sweet Potato Brownies With Crushed Almonds

Prep Time: 10 minutes|Cook Time: 20 mins| Total Time: 30 mins| Difficulty: Easy

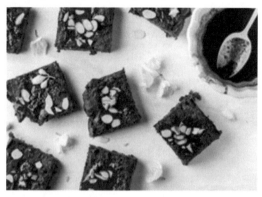

### Ingredients:

- ½ cup mashed sweet potato
- 1 tbsp. peanut butter
- ¼ cup almond flour
- 2 tbsp. cocoa powder
- one medium egg
- ¼ tsp baking powder
- 1 tsp maple syrup
- ¼ tsp vanilla extract
- 2 tbsp dark chocolate chips
- Pinch of cinnamon powder
- 5g crushed almonds

### Instructions:

1. Combine mashed sweet potato, peanut butter, egg, and maple syrup in a bowl. Mix the remaining ingredients until the batter is well combined. Fold in dark chocolate chips and crushed almonds
2. Preheat oven to 175 C. Grease the baking dish with 1 tsp extra virgin olive oil.
3. Place the batter in the prepared baking dish and bake for 20-25 mins.
4. Serve immediately.

Total calories: 615 Carbohydrates: 56g Proteins: 21g Fat: 36g

## 1. Spinach Mushroom Lasagna with ricotta cheese

Prep Time: 15 minutes| Cook Time: 35 mins| Total Time: 50 mins| Difficulty: Easy

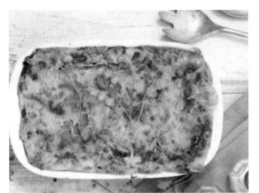

**Ingredients:**

- 6 whole wheat lasagna sheets, boiled
- 1 cup fresh baby spinach leaves, chopped
- ¼ cup mushrooms, sliced
- ½ zucchini, peeled and grated
- ½ cup ricotta cheese
- ½ cup parmesan cheese
- ¼ tsp turmeric powder
- ¼ tsp dried basil
- ¼ tsp dried oregano
- 1 tbsp extra virgin olive oil
- 1 tbsp parsley

**Instructions:**

1. Preheat oven to 190 C.
2. Boil lasagna sheets as per package instructions. Set them aside.
3. Heat olive oil in a non-stick pan & add minced garlic, chopped spinach, grated zucchini, and all the spices mentioned.
4. Cook for 5 minutes until this mixture becomes a smooth paste.
5. Add marinara sauce to a baking dish and place two sheets of lasagna on top.
6. Repeat the layer, top it with chili flakes and parsley, and bake for 20-25 minutes.

Total calories: 955  Carbohydrates: 105g  Proteins: 47g  Fat: 41g

## 2. Turkey and Rolled Oats Meatballs

Prep Time: 10 minutes| Cook Time: 20 mins| Total Time: 30 mins| Difficulty: Easy

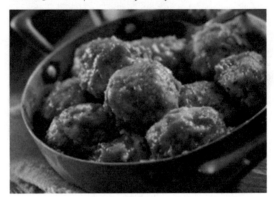

**Ingredients:**

- 200 g ground turkey
- ¼ cup rolled oats
- ½ small carrot, peeled and grated
- ½ small zucchini, peeled and grated
- ¼ small onion, chopped
- ¼ tsp garlic powder
- one medium egg
- 1 tbsp Worcestershire sauce
- ¼ tsp turmeric powder
- Salt and black pepper as per taste
- 1 tbsp olive oil

**Instructions:**

1. Combine turkey, rolled oats, grated carrots, zucchini, and all the remaining ingredients in a bowl. Mix well until well combined.
2. Using your hands, shape this mixture into meatballs about 1 inch each.
3. Heat olive oil in a nonstick pan. Add the meatballs and cook for 3-4 minutes on each side.
4. Preheat oven to 190 C. Shift them in a baking tray and bake for 10-15 minutes until they get a brown and crispy texture.
5. Serve immediately.

Total calories: 568  Carbohydrates: 25g  Proteins: 67g  Fat: 20g

## 3. Black beans & sweet potato tacos

Prep Time: 15 minutes| Cook Time: 25 mins| Total Time: 40 mins| Difficulty: Easy

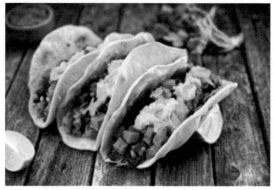

**Ingredients:**

- Sweet potatoes:
- One small, sweet potato, peeled and diced
- 1 tsp olive oil
- ¼ tsp paprika powder
- Pinch of sea salt
- Black beans:
- ½ cup canned black beans
- ½ small onion, chopped
- ¼ tsp ground cumin
- 1 tsp lime juice
- Sea salt & black pepper as per taste
- 1 tbsp olive oil
- Fresh cilantro leaves (for topping)

**Instructions:**

1. Preheat oven to 200 C.
2. Add olive oil, a pinch of sea salt, and paprika powder to the cubes of sweet potatoes and bake them for 20 minutes until golden brown.
3. Prepare the black beans, add all the ingredients mentioned, and mix them well.
4. Now heat the tortilla wrap, arrange the layers of sweet potato and black beans, and fold it.
5. Top it with fresh cilantro leaves & serve immediately.

Total calories: 305  Carbohydrates: 36g     Proteins: 10g     Fat: 14g

## 4. Chicken Wrap with Yogurt Sauce

Prep Time: 15 minutes| Cook Time: 20 mins| Total Time: 35 mins| Difficulty: Easy

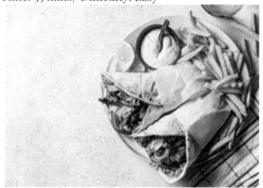

**Ingredients:**

- Chicken:
- one boneless, skinless chicken breast
- ½ tsp ground turmeric
- ¼ tsp of Sumac or lemon zest
- ¼ tsp ground coriander
- Wrap:
- one whole-grain or spinach tortilla wrap
- 1/8 avocado, sliced
- ¼ cup mixed greens
- ¼ cup purple cabbage
- 3 tbsp yogurt

**Instructions:**

1. Marinate your chicken with all the chicken ingredients for 2 hours. Coat the chicken well.
2. Cook the marinated chicken in a non-stick pan for 5-7 minutes for each side until the color of the chicken is golden brown and the meat is fully cooked.
3. Whisk in all the yogurt sauce ingredients and prepare the delicious sauce. Taste and adjust the seasonings accordingly.
4. Now heat the whole-grain tortilla wrap and layer it with veggies. Top it off with the cooked boneless chicken.
5. Pour the yogurt sauce over the chicken and fold the wraps from both sides.

Total calories: 308  Carbohydrates: 20g     Proteins: 26g     Fat: 16g

## 5. Whole-Wheat Spaghetti

Prep Time: 10 minutes| Cook Time: 15 mins| Total Time: 25 mins| Difficulty: Easy

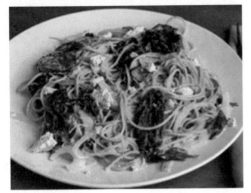

**Ingredients:**
- 2 oz whole wheat spaghetti
- 1 tbsp Pesto Infused Olive Oil
- ¼ cup fresh spinach leaves
- 2 cloves of garlic
- ¼ cup sun-dried tomatoes
- ¼ cup spinach
- 1 tbsp pine nuts
- 1 tsp lime zest
- Salt and pepper
- Fresh parsley (garnish)

**Instructions:**

1. Add water to a large pot and 1 tsp salt. Please bring it to a boil.

2. Drain the pasta and set aside, but reserve ¼ cup of pasta water.

3. While the pasta is boiling, roast the pine nuts in a small dry pan for 2-3 minutes until fragrant and changing color. Remove from the pan, and set the nuts aside.

4. Add peso-infused olive oil to the same pan, sauté garlic and sun-dried tomatoes for 2 minutes.

5. Add the cooked spaghetti and reserved pasta water to the pan.

6. Place the cooked spaghetti on a serving plate and top with roasted pine nuts and fresh parsley.

Total calories: 228  Carbohydrates: 24g    Proteins: 7g    Fat: 14g

## 6. Spicy Shrimp Coconut Milk Curry

Prep Time: 12 minutes| Cook Time: 18 mins| Total Time: 30 mins| Difficulty: Easy

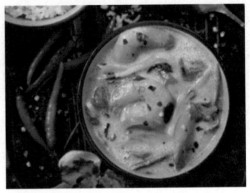

**Ingredients:**
- 6-8 peeled shrimp
- 1 tbsp coconut oil
- ½ onion
- two garlic cloves
- ¼ cup cherry tomatoes
- ½ tbsp grated ginger
- 1 tbsp curry powder
- ¼ tsp Shichimi Togarashi or any other chili spices such as chili flakes
- Pinch of salt and pepper
- ½ tsp turmeric
- ¼ cup coconut milk
- Fresh cilantro (garnish)

**Instructions:**

1. Heat coconut oil in a pan and saute onion in it. Then add garlic and ginger and cook for 2 mins.

2. Then add the spices and mix well. Cook for another minute for the fragrance and flavor.

3. add the shrimp to the pan, cooking each side for 2 minutes.

4. Next, add coconut milk and cherry tomatoes. Simmer it for 4-5 minutes.

5. Once the sauce thickens, your dinner will be served. Transfer it to the serving plate and garnish with fresh cilantro. Serve with jasmine rice or naan & enjoy.

Total calories: 323  Carbohydrates: 14g    Proteins: 9g    Fat: 27g

# 7. Broccoli & Cheddar Soup

Prep Time: 10 minutes| Cook Time: 20 mins| Total
Time: 30 mins| Difficulty: Easy

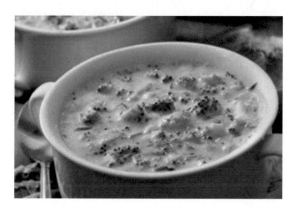

## Ingredients:

- 1 cup broccoli florets
- 1 tbsp avocado oil
- ½ small onion
- 1 tbsp chickpea flour
- ½ cup low-sodium vegetable broth
- ½ cup unsweetened almond milk
- ¼ tsp turmeric
- ¼ tsp Dijon mustard
- 1 tsp truffle honey
- Salt and pepper

## Instructions:

1. Heat coconut oil in a pan and sauté the aromatics for 3-4 minutes. Then add chickpea flour and combine well.
2. Then add vegetable broth, stirring continuously to prevent lumps. Add broccoli florets and simmer the mixture for 10 minutes.
3. Transfer this soup to a blender and blend to your preferred texture. Then, please return it to the pot.
4. Then add almond milk and spices. Taste and adjust the seasonings. Stir continuously for a creamy soup.
5. Transfer to the serving bowl and serve immediately.

Total calories: 264  Carbohydrates:
28g        Proteins: 6g      Fat: 18g

# 8. Vegan Detox Spring Rolls

Prep Time: 15 minutes| Cook Time: 10 mins| Total
Time: 25 mins| Difficulty: Easy

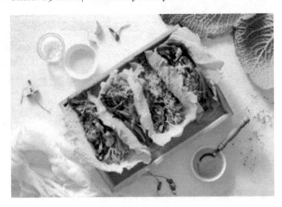

## Ingredients:

- 3-4 rice paper wrapper
- ¼ cup cooked quinoa
- ¼ cup alfalfa sprouts
- ¼ cup sliced carrots
- ¼ cup sliced bell peppers
- 1 tbsp pickled ginger
- 1 tbsp fresh mint leaves
- Peanut Sauce
- 2 tbsp peanut butter
- 1 tbsp tamari sauce
- 1 tsp lime juice
- 1 tsp maple syrup
- ½ tsp grated ginger
- ¼ tsp sesame oil
- ¼ tsp red pepper

## Instructions:

1. Add warm water in a shallow dish and submerge a rice paper wrapper for 12 seconds until it gets soft and flexible.
2. Add quinoa, sprouts, and veggies in the middle of the wrapper.
3. Fold the edges of the wrapper over the filling, then roll tightly from the bottom to form a compact cylinder. Continue this process with the remaining wrappers and fillings.
4. Make the Thai peanut sauce by whisking together all the ingredients in a bowl.
5. Arrange the rolls on your serving plate and serve with Thai sauce.

Total calories: 187   Carbohydrates:
33g  Proteins: 5g   Fat: 4g

# HASSLE FREE ANTI-INFLAMMATORY DIET COOKBOOK

## HELP US GROW WITH YOUR REVIEW!

**WE'D LOVE YOUR FEEDBACK!**

THANK YOU FOR CHOOSING THIS BOOK AS PART OF YOUR HEALTH JOURNEY. YOUR FEEDBACK MEANS THE WORLD TO US! IF YOU'VE ENJOYED THE RECIPES AND FOUND THE INFORMATION HELPFUL, PLEASE CONSIDER LEAVING A POSITIVE REVIEW. SIMPLY SCAN THE QR CODE BELOW TO SHARE YOUR THOUGHTS.

YOUR REVIEW HELPS US REACH MORE PEOPLE AND CONTINUE SPREADING THE MESSAGE OF HEALTHY LIVING.

## THANK YOU FOR YOUR SUPPORT!

# Building a Family Meal Plan on Budget

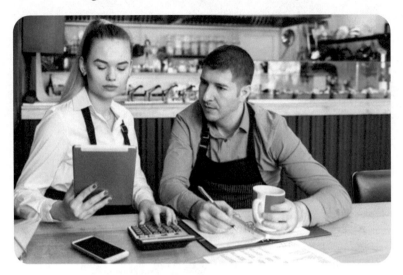

Preparing a family meal plan on a tight budget is fun, and every family should challenge themselves to do it because it is effective, efficient, and beneficial in the long run. Making a diet meal plan and preparing healthy and tasty food without overspending is always possible. Here are some steps and things to consider when planning a family meal that will not break the bank.

### Assess Your Budget

Knowing how much you intend to spend on groceries each week or month is the best way to start. Understanding the amount of food money each week enables you to cook meals within your allotted budget. Divide the budget into portions covering proteins, vegetables, grains, and snacks. In this way, one can apply the funds as required and is not stuck with purchasing items that fall into the depleted budget category.

### Cost-Effective Shopping Tips

If you want to maximize your grocery budget, implement some economical strategies. For example, it's advisable to purchase a large package of low-priced foods, such as rice, pasta, or canned meals. Some grocery stores offer bulk purchase discounts, and taking advantage of these bulk discounts helps prepare a lot amount of meals.

Opting for seasonal foods is a savvy move, as they pack a punch in terms of health benefits. Freshly harvested vegetables and fruits, having not been stored for long periods, are more nutritious and easier on the wallet than their out-of-season counterparts. Keep in mind that the out-of-season counterparts usually need to be shipped from a substantial distance, which only raises the cost.

## Meal Planning Techniques

Weekly meal planning is critical to curbing impulse purchases and avoiding frequent last-minute shopping trips. By dedicating time each week to assessing your pantry and fridge, you can plan your meals using existing ingredients, minimizing the need for additional purchases.

After you are through with your meal plan for the week, take your time to prepare a detailed shopping list, which will come in handy. This will help you resist the so-called 'mid-week munchies' and greatly assist you in only buying what is necessary for the whole week. You should also do a check on weekly sales, preferably before finalizing your meal plan. Good sales can stretch your food budget to the maximum. Also, try portioning the meals and cooking them in significant quantities so they can be reheated and eaten later. This helps avoid the regular order of expensive take out during the busy working days, providing you with the convenience of ready-to-eat meals.

## Budget-Friendly Ingredients

It takes cautious management to ensure that your food is cheap because the cost of the food ingredients forms a large part of the total budget. Products such as beans, lentils, and rice are good examples of reasonable anti-inflammatory foods that can be used in many healthy recipes and that contain good nutritional value.

Consumers need to identify excellent and affordable cuts of meat that, if properly cooked, are as tasty as the highly-priced ones. For protein, go for the cheaper parts of meat that are still as good, such as thighs, shoulder, and beef. These foods are affordable, and most importantly, they offer significant health benefits to the human body, reassuring you that you can eat healthily on a budget.

## Resource Management

This strategy will help reduce wastage and ensure your groceries last longer than expected. The first step to getting started is to sort out all items stored in your pantry and the fridge to ensure they can be easily seen. Stack close-to-expiration foods in more accessible positions while applying the 'FIFO- first in, first out' principle. Also, it's unwise to trash edible food, so get creative and convert your leftovers into another tasty meal. For instance, the uneaten roasted vegetables can be used to prepare a frittata and leftover cooked chicken can be used to make sandwiches or salads.

# Fun Cooking Activities to Do with Kids

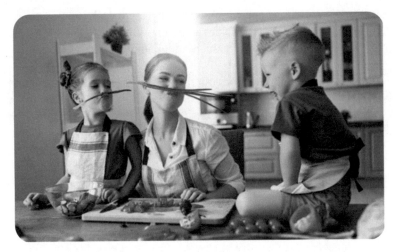

Cooking is an essential survival role that all should become familiar with. While men and women should know how to cook, bringing your kids into the kitchen and teaching them the basics would be great. Preparing food with kids is a great idea to make a child interested in the meals they eat. Moreover, it is an easy and entertaining way to unite the whole family. But I assure you it goes beyond just coming up with meals; it's an opportunity to bond with loved ones, explore new culinary skills, and discover the richness of various cultures through the universal language of food. Inviting your children into the kitchen ensures they develop a love for cooking, and they feel happy and proud when they make something tasty using their little fingers.

### Cooking Classes at Home

Are you bored with washing spoons, forks, and other utensils? Why not turn your kitchen into a classroom and let your kids learn how to prepare different meals independently? Tiny hands, significant impact! Give your children a healthy and educational break from their cell phones by arranging a sushi-making class and teaching your tiny chefs the art of making dough, kneading, and rolling. Similarly, creating homemade pasta with kids will be an unlimited fun project. Such engaging cooking classes will help your kids learn simple recipe preparation. They will also get familiar with foods from different cultures.

### Theme Nights

Engaging your children in cooking can be challenging, but it becomes easier when you do things in ways that they love. Organize different cultural food theme nights for your kids, where they can immerse themselves in various traditions. For example, organize a Mexican evening for kids and explain how you make tacos, quesadillas, or guacamole. You can set the table with traditional decorations and play traditional music to add more fun. Having a pizza party night can be another fun and tasty approach to involving your kids in cooking in a fun way. They can make their dough and even select the toppings of their choice

63

**Food Art**

Food art is an excellent way to encourage kids to eat more appealing, healthy foods. Have your kids prepare fruit plates or funky faces on pizza using components such as peppers, olives, and tomatoes. You can also use cookie cutters and let them create attractive appearances for fruits, sandwiches, and other dishes. This activity is a great way to encourage them to eat more fruits and vegetables whenever possible.

Involving your children in cooking is a beautiful way to impart valuable life lessons to them and create memories that last a lifetime! So, wear your aprons and get ready for a remarkable culinary journey with your family.

## Educating your Family on Eating Healthy

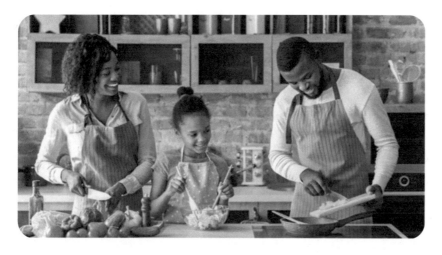

The world we live in today is no less than a global village.From eating raw vegetables and fruit and eating hunted animals to exploring the world of fast food, seafood, and seasonal food, we've come a long way! Unfortunately, together with this new sophistication came the impending challenges of increased health problems, including Diabetes, Obesity, Hypertension, & Cardiovascular diseases. According to the World Health Organization (WHO), the obesity rate has more than doubled since 1990, with 1 in 8 people in the world living with obesity in 2022.

Therefore, we must take our health and nutrition very seriously and educate ourselves and our families on the benefits of eating a balanced, notoriously healthy diet.

**Engaging Discussions**

We must engage in interactive discussions with our parents & children and emphasize having a balanced diet with a proper eating schedule. Children, especially, should be advised not to depend too much on junk foods, as various types of research have proved that lack of proper nutrition in children does hinder intellectual and physical growth as they fail to achieve their full potential.

**Role Modelling**

The haphazard and excessive intake of sugars, oil, and spices can result in various metabolic and cardiovascular diseases in adults and early. Therefore, parents must give special attention to their children's caloric intake and eating schedule. Adding exercise and walking to daily life significantly reduces the risk of diseases and keeps your body healthy. The adults have an essential role to play here, as children often learn from what they observe. As an adult, you are responsible for keeping your family healthy and sound. Make sure you eat, sleep, and wake up on time. Take the children with you for a walk. Please encourage them to engage in healthy extra-curricular activities. Sports provide a boost to both the body and the mind.

**Nutritional Literacy**

Another critical factor that can help you maintain a healthy lifestyle is Nutritional literacy. You must understand your daily caloric, protein, carbohydrate, and fat requirements. You should know and teach your family to read food labels and realize the calories a packet of chips provides per serving. Encouraging Independence

Lastly, we need to invite our kids to participate in grocery shopping and empower them to make healthy choices. This will boost their confidence, excite them about adding healthy items to their eating schedule, and teach them to appreciate their health. This way, we can ensure that we and our family have a rich, healthy lifestyle and avoid the risks of diseases.

# CHAPTER 4

## DIETARY RESTRICTIONS AND MODIFICATIONS

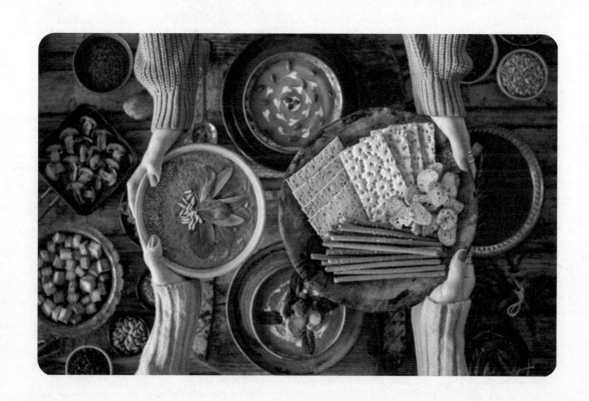

## 1. Oatmeal zucchini pancakes

Prep Time: 10 minutes| Cook Time: 15mins| Total Time: 25 mins| Difficulty: Easy

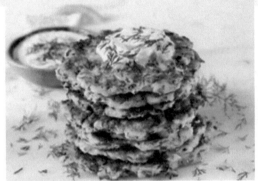

### Ingredients:

- One medium zucchini, peeled and grated
- ¼ cup whole wheat flour
- ¼ cup oats flour
- 1/3 cup spring water
- One medium egg
- ½ tsp ground cumin
- ¼ cup cilantro leaves
- 1 tbsp olive oil
- For the green sauce:
- ¼ cup Greek yogurt
- ½ tsp parsley
- 1 tsp lime juice
- Pinch of black pepper

### Instructions:

1. Add grated zucchini, sea salt, and black pepper to a bowl. Mix well and let it sit for 10 minutes.
2. Prepare the green sauce by mixing Greek yogurt, lime juice, parsley leaves, salt, and black pepper.
3. Now prepare the batter by adding egg, whole wheat flour, oat flour, cilantro leaves, and water to the zucchini mixture.
4. Heat a non-stick pan on medium heat and grease it with olive oil.
5. Cook for 2-3 minutes each side. Repeat until all the batter is finished.
6. Serve warm with the green sauce.

Total calories: 462 Carbohydrates: 46g     Proteins 22g     Fat: 22g

## 2. Millet porridge with roasted flax seeds & blueberries

Prep Time: 5 minutes| Cook Time: 25 mins| Total Time: 30 mins| Difficulty: Easy

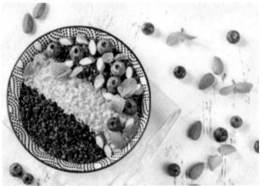

### Ingredients:

- ½ cup millet, washed & rinsed
- 1 cup approx. 240 ml spring water
- 1 tbsp roasted flax seeds
- Pinch of cardamom powder
- ¼ tsp cinnamon powder
- 1 tsp manuka honey
- For the topping:
- ¼ cup fresh blueberries
- 1 tbsp roasted flaxseeds

### Instructions:

1. Add rinsed millet, cardamom powder, cinnamon powder, and water to a saucepan and boil over medium heat. Gradually reduce the heat to low and let it cook for 15-20 minutes until all the water is absorbed.
2. In a separate pan, roast the flax seeds for 2-3 minutes and set them aside.
3. Transfer the cooked millet to a serving bowl. Top it with roasted flax seeds, fresh blueberries, and a drizzle of manuka honey.
4. Serve immediately.

Total calories: 475 Carbohydrates: 81g     Proteins: 10g     Fat: 12.8g

## 3. Lemon & Rosemary Roasted Chickpeas

Prep Time: 10 minutes| Cook Time: 20 mins| Total Time: 30 mins| Difficulty: Easy

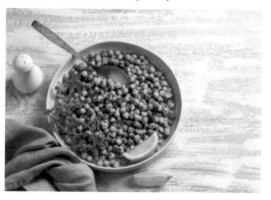

### Ingredients:

- ½ cup cooked canned chickpeas (Garbanzo beans)
- 1 tsp lime juice
- 1 tsp extra virgin olive oil
- ¼ tsp fresh rosemary, chopped
- Sea salt and paper as per taste
- Pinch of turmeric powder
- 1 tbsp cilantro leaves (for topping)

### Instructions:

1. Preheat oven to 190 C.
2. In a bowl, add cooked chickpeas, lime juice, chopped rosemary, a pinch of turmeric powder, sea salt, and pepper. Mix well.
3. Transfer them to a baking tray greased with olive oil. Bake for 20 minutes until they get crunchy and crispy.
4. Serve immediately.

Total calories: 179 Carbohydrates: 22.1g Proteins: 7.33g Fat: 6.53

## 4. Figs & Grapes Salad with Cottage Cheese

Prep Time: 10 minutes| Cook Time: 0 mins| Total Time: 10 mins| Difficulty: Easy

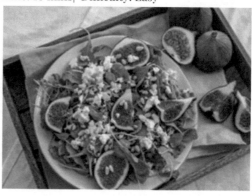

### Ingredients:

- Three fresh figs, washed & cut in quarters
- ½ cup red or black grapes, washed & halved
- ¼ tsp cinnamon powder
- ¼ cup low-sodium cottage cheese
- 1 tsp manuka honey
- 5 g walnuts, crushed

### Instructions:

1. In a bowl, assemble the quartered figs and halved grapes.
2. Layer cottage cheese over it. Sprinkle cinnamon powder and mix well. Add crushed walnuts for an extra crunch. Drizzle manuka honey over it.
3. Serve immediately.

Total calories: 261 Carbohydrates: 49g Proteins: 9.5g Fat: 6.1g

## 5. Grilled Salmon & Lime Roasted vegetable skewers

Prep Time: 10 minutes| Cook Time: 20 mins|
Total Time: 30 mins| Difficulty: Easy

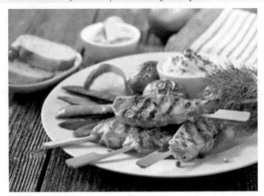

### Ingredients:

- For the salmon:
- One salmon fillet approx. 4-6 oz
- ½ tsp. turmeric powder
- 1 tbsp lime juice
- 1 tbsp extra virgin olive oil
- Sea salt as per taste
- For the roasted veggies:
- ½ red bell pepper, squared cut
- ½ small red onion, cubed
- ½ yellow bell pepper
- 1 tsp lime juice
- 1 tbsp parsley (for topping)

### Instructions:

1. Marinate the salmon fillet with salt, pepper, turmeric powder, lime juice,garlic powder, pepper and salt for 15 minutes.
2. Grease a nonstick pan with olive oil and grill the salmon for almost 4-5 minutes on each side.
3. Now grill the squared and cubed onion and bell peppers in the same pan for 2 minutes on high flame.
4. Arrange the roasted vegetables and grilled salmon in skewers.
5. Serve immediately.

Total calories: 403 Carbohydrates:12.3g
Proteins:26.7g Fat: 29.3g

## 6. Egg-Fried Rice with Stir Fry Broccoli & Carrot

Prep Time: 10 minutes| Cook Time: 20 mins|
Total Time: 30 mins| Difficulty: Medium

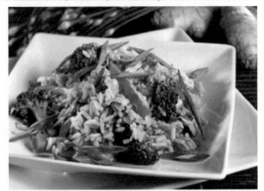

### Ingredients:

- For the egg fried rice:
- ½ cup cooked brown rice
- One medium egg (slightly beaten)
- ¼ cup green onions
- One clove of garlic, crushed
- 1 tsp Bragg Coconut aminos or ½ tsp of Soy sauce
- 1 tsp Worcestershire sauce
- 1 tsp avocado oil
- 1 tsp balsamic vinegar
- Salt and pepper as per taste
- For the Stir-fry broccoli and carrots:
- ½ cup broccoli florets
- ½ cup carrot, peeled and grated

### Instructions:

1. Add 1 tsp extra virgin olive oil to a saucepan. Stir-fry broccoli florets and grated carrots on high flame for 2-3 minutes.
2. Heat avocado oil and sauté crushed garlic in the same pan for over 1 minute. Transfer the beaten egg and scramble it until it is fully cooked.
3. Add the cooked brown rice, coconut aminos, Worcestershire sauce, balsamic vinegar and toss well. Sprinkle salt and pepper to taste. Add green onion and let it cook for 1 minute.
4. Transfer them to a serving plate and serve immediately.

Total calories: 391 Carbohydrates: 40g Proteins: 10g Fat: 15.2g

## 7. Grilled Chicken With Roasted Green Beans & Sweet Potatoes

Prep Time: 10 minutes| Cook Time: 20 mins|
Total Time: 30 mins| Difficulty: Easy

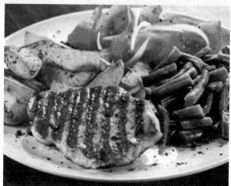

### Ingredients:

- For the egg fried rice:
- 200 g chicken breast
- 1 tbsp extra virgin olive oil
- ¼ tsp garlic powder
- 1/8 tsp ginger powder
- 1 tsp Worcestershire sauce
- For the roasted green beans and sweet potatoes:
- 100 g green beans, trimmed
- one small, sweet potato cut into wedges
- Salt and black pepper as per taste

### Instructions:

1. Marinate the chicken breast for 20 minutes with garlic, ginger powder, fresh thyme, dried oregano, olive oil, lime juice, Worcestershire sauce, salt, and pepper.
2. Preheat the oven to 200 C.
3. Place the sweet potato and green beans on a baking tray seasoned with salt and black pepper and bake them for 15-20 minutes.
4. Meanwhile, grease the grill pan with olive oil over medium heat and grill the marinated chicken breast.
5. Transfer the grilled chicken to a serving plate and assemble the roasted green beans and sweet potato on top of it.
6. Serve immediately.

Total calories: 729    Carbohydrates: 36.3g    Proteins:66.5g    Fat: 35.4g

## 8. Almond & coconut energy balls

Prep Time: 15 minutes| Cook Time:0 mins|
Total Time: 15 mins| Difficulty: Easy

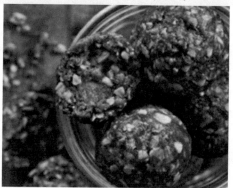

### Ingredients:

- 4 tbsp almond flour
- 2 tbsp shredded coconut
- 2 tbsp almond butter
- 1 tbsp coconut oil
- Pinch of cinnamon
- Pinch of cardamon powder
- 1 tbsp acacia or raw honey
- 1 tsp sesame seeds powder

### Instructions:

1. Combine all the dry ingredients: almond flour, shredded coconut, cinnamon, cardamon powder, and sesame seeds powder.
2. Add all wet ingredients: almond butter, coconut oil, and honey. Mix well until it becomes thick and dough-like. If the mixture is too dry, add some coconut oil to adjust.
3. Roll this mixture with your hands and shape it into small balls. This mixture will give you 5-6 energy balls.
4. Add shredded coconut to a separate plate and toss over the energy balls in it one by one to evenly spread the coconut coating.
5. Serve immediately.

Total calories: 666  Carbohydrates: 34g    Proteins: 15g    Fat: 56.5g

# 1. Dairy-Free Almond & Raspberry Smoothie

Prep Time: 10 minutes| Cook Time: 0 mins| Total Time: 10 mins| Difficulty: Easy

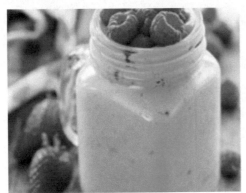

## Ingredients:

- ½ cup fresh or frozen raspberries
- ½ small banana
- ½ cup almond or soy milk
- ¼ cup almond yogurt
- 1 tsp almond butter
- 1 tsp hemp seeds
- 5g almonds

## Instructions:

1. Blend all ingredients quickly until you achieve a smooth and creamy consistency.
2. If the smoothie is too thick, add half a cup of almond milk to get the desired consistency.
3. Transfer the smoothie into a glass and garnish with fresh raspberries!

Total calories: 303   Carbohydrates: 29g
Proteins: 9.7g      Fat: 18.4g

# 2. Blueberry Coconut Smoothie Bowl

Prep Time: 10 minutes| Cook Time: 0 mins| Total Time: 10 mins| Difficulty: Easy

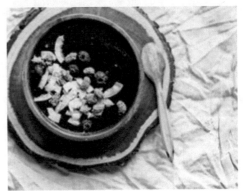

## Ingredients:

- ½ cup blueberries
- ½ cup coconut yogurt
- ½ small banana
- ½ cup approx. 120 ml almond milk or any plant-based milk of your choice
- 1 tsp almond butter
- For topping:
- 1 tbsp shredded coconut
- ¼ cup mixed berries
- 1 tsp chia seeds soaked in water for 10-15 minutes

## Instructions:

1. Blend blueberries, coconut yogurt, almond milk, and banana until you achieve a smooth consistency.
2. Transfer this smoothie mixture into a bowl and garnish with shredded coconut, some berries, and chia seeds. Refrigerate for 30 minutes before serving.

Total calories: 442   Carbohydrates: 43.6g Proteins: 9.8g      Fat: 29.7g

## 3. Cashew Cream Cheese Spread with Garlic Bread Toast

Prep Time: 10 minutes| Cook Time: 4 mins|
Total Time: 14 mins| Difficulty: Easy

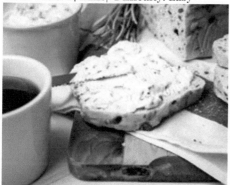

### Ingredients:

- ½ cup cashews, soaked for 4 hours
- 1 tbsp lime juice
- 1 tbsp apple cider vinegar or balsamic vinegar
- Salt as per taste
- 2-3 tbsp water
- 1 tbsp parsley or dill, as per your choice
- For garlic bread:
- 1-2 cloves of garlic, crushed
- 1 tbsp olive oil
- Two slices of whole-wheat bread

### Instructions:

1. Blend the soaked cashews, lime juice, apple cider vinegar, and water until smooth and creamy. Add 1 tbsp parsley to give the cashew cream cheese extra flavor.
2. Mix crushed garlic and olive oil in a small bowl and brush it over the whole wheat bread slices.
3. Toast the bread slices for 4 minutes on each side and spread cashew cream cheese.
4. Serve immediately.

Total calories: 647    Carbohydrates: 47.2g    Proteins: 16.5g    Fat: 46g

## 4. Overnight Oatmeal and Chia Chocolate Pudding

Prep Time: 10 minutes| Cook Time: 0 mins|
Total Time: 10 mins| Difficulty: Easy

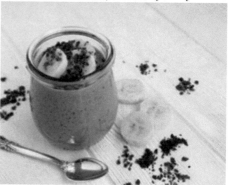

### Ingredients:

- ¼ cup rolled oats
- 2 tbsp chia seeds
- ½ cup oat milk or almond milk
- 2 tbsp cacao powder
- ¼ tsp cinnamon powder
- ¼ tsp vanilla extract
- For topping:
- ½ sliced banana
- Crushed dark chocolate

### Instructions:

1. Combine all the ingredients in a jar. Cover the jar and refrigerate for 4 hours or overnight until a thick pudding-like consistency forms.
2. Top it with sliced banana, crushed dark chocolate, and mixed nuts.

Total calories: 450  Carbohydrates: 74g    Proteins: 11.6g    Fat: 16g

## 5. Cashew Yogurt Raspberry Parfait

Prep Time: 10 minutes| Chill Time: 30 mins| Total Time: 40 mins| Difficulty: Easy

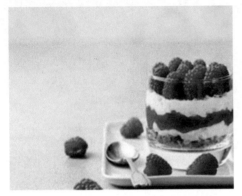

### Ingredients:

- ½ cup cashew or almond yogurt
- 1 tbsp raw honey
- For topping:
- ½ cup raspberries
- 5g cashews or any other nuts
- 5g almonds
- 2 tbsp granola

### Instructions:

1. Add ¼ cup yogurt to a jar. Add ½ tbsp honey and 1 tbsp granola over it. Add ¼ cup of raspberries.
2. Repeat the layers.
3. Garnish with chopped nuts on top and some raspberries.
4. Refrigerate it for 30 minutes before serving.

Total calories: 323 Carbohydrates: 45.6g Proteins: 8.1g Fat: 16g

## 6. Almond Oatmeal Wrap with Banana Topping

Prep Time: 10 minutes| Chill Time: 30 mins| Total Time: 40 mins| Difficulty: Easy

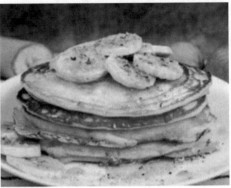

### Ingredients:

- ¼ cup oat flour
- ¼ cup almond flour
- ¼ cup almond milk or soy milk
- ¼ tsp baking powder
- Pinch of cinnamon powder
- ¼ tsp vanilla extract
- For topping:
- ½ sliced banana
- 5g crushed almonds

### Instructions:

1. In a bowl, combine all the dry ingredients.
2. Add almond milk to all the dry ingredients until a thick and smooth paste is formed.
3. Grease the pan with olive oil, spread the mixture evenly with the back of a spoon, and give it a round shape.
4. Cook for 3 minutes on each side until a golden-brown color is achieved.
4. Serve immediately and garnish with sliced banana.

Total calories: 369 Carbohydrates: 39g Proteins: 9.9g Fat: 17g

## 7. Dairy-free Blueberry Banana Smoothie

Prep Time: 10 minutes| Cook Time: 0 mins|
Total Time: 10 mins| Difficulty: Easy

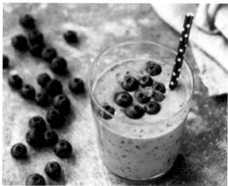

**Ingredients:**

- ½ cup blueberries
- one small banana, sliced
- ½ cup oat milk
- ¼ cup oat yogurt
- 5g pecans
- 1 tsp flax seeds

**Instructions:**

1. Combine all the ingredients.
2. Blend all ingredients at high speed until you achieve a smooth and creamy consistency.
3. If the smoothie is too thick, add half a cup of more oat milk to adjust the consistency.
4. Serve immediately.

Total calories: 258   Carbohydrates: 49g
Proteins: 4.5g      Fat: 7g

## 8. Broccoli & Strawberry Salad with Almond Yogurt Dressing

Prep Time: 15 minutes| Cook Time: 0 mins|
Total Time: 15 mins| Difficulty: Easy

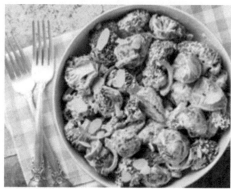

**Ingredients:**

- ½ cup broccoli florets
- ½ cup strawberries, halved
- ½ small red onion, peeled and chopped
- ½ cup arugula, chopped
- ¼ cup chopped almond
- For almond yogurt dressing:
- ¼ cup almond yogurt
- Salt and pepper as per taste
- 1 tsp lemon juice

**Instructions:**

1. Combine broccoli florets, halved strawberries, chopped red onion, and arugula in a bowl.
2. Mix almond yogurt dressing with almond yogurt, lime juice, salt and pepper. Mix well until it forms a smooth paste.
3. Toss the dressing with the salad and garnish with chopped almonds.
4. Serve immediately.

Total calories: 119   Carbohydrates: 23g   Proteins: 4.7g      Fat: 2.1g

## 1. Mixed Fruit Salad Bowl

Prep Time: 10 minutes| Cook Time: 0 mins|
Total Time: 10 mins| Difficulty: Easy

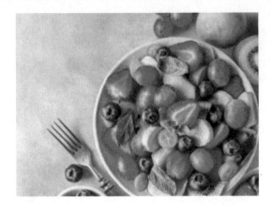

**Ingredients:**

- One small kiwi, peeled and sliced
- ½ cup strawberries, halved
- ½ small peach, cubed
- ¼ cup red grapes
- ¼ cup blueberries
- one kumquat, sliced (Optional) or ½ orange juice
- 1 tsp fresh lime
- ¼ tsp fresh ground black pepper
- Few fresh mint leaves

**Instructions:**

1. Combine all the fruit in a bowl.
2. Add lime juice and black pepper over the salad. Mix well. Garnish with some fresh mint leaves.
3. Serve immediately.

Total calories: 152   Carbohydrates: 35g
Proteins: 2.6g      Fat: 1g

## 2. Lime Infused Watermelon Cold-pressed Juice

Prep Time: 10 minutes| Cook Time: 0 mins|
Total Time: 10 mins| Difficulty: Easy

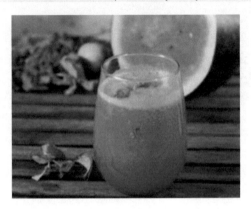

**Ingredients:**

- 2 cups watermelon, cubed and seeds removed
- 1 tsp lime juice
- Fresh mint leaves

**Instructions:**

1. Turn on the cold press juicer machine. Add cubed watermelon to it.
2. Allow the juicer to extract the juice properly.
3. Transfer the juice into a serving glass, add lime juice, and garnish with fresh mint leaves.
4. Serve immediately.

Total calories: 92   Carbohydrates: 23.5g   Proteins: 1.8g      Fat: 0.2g

## 3. Shredded Chicken Salad with Tangerine

Prep Time: 10 minutes| Cook Time: 0 mins| Total Time: 10 mins| Difficulty: Easy

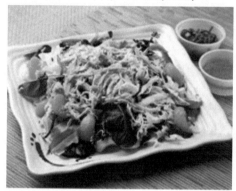

**Ingredients:**

- 1 cup shredded chicken
- 1 tangerine, peeled and segmented
- ¼ cup purple cabbage
- ¼ cup lettuce leaves, chopped
- 5g crushed walnuts
- 1 tsp lime juice
- 1 tsp apple cider vinegar
- Fresh ground black pepper as per taste

**Instructions:**

1. If you don't have pre-cooked shredded chicken, boil 200 g chicken breast in 2 cups water for 20-25 minutes and let cool.
2. Combine all the ingredients in a bowl. Add lime juice, apple cider vinegar, and black pepper. Mix well. Sprinkle crushed walnuts on top.
3. Serve immediately.

Total calories: 334    Carbohydrates: 16.5g    Proteins: 44.9g    Fat: 8.4g

## 4. Chia Seed Pudding with Pomegranate Seeds

Prep Time: 10 minutes| Chill Time: 4 hrs| Total Time: 4 hrs 10 mins| Difficulty: Easy

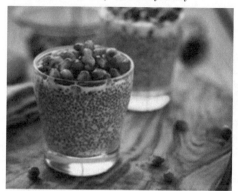

**Ingredients:**

- ½ cup almond milk
- 2.5 tbsp chia seeds
- ¼ tsp cinnamon powder
- honey to taste
- 2-3 drops of vanilla extract
- For topping:
- ¼ cup pomegranate seeds
- 5g crushed almonds

**Instructions:**

1. Add almond milk, chia seeds, cinnamon, cardamom powder, and honey to a bowl. Stir it well so that no lumps form. Cover and refrigerate for 3-4 hours.
2. Add pomegranate seeds and crushed almonds on top.
3. Serve immediately.

Total calories: 267  Carbohydrates: 35.4g    Proteins: 7.5g    Fat: 14.2g

## 5. Low-Sodium White Bean Soup with Carrot & Celery

Prep Time: 10 minutes| Cook Time: 90 mins|
Total Time: 100 mins| Difficulty: Medium

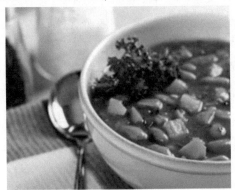

### Ingredients:

- ½ cup white beans (preferably navy or cannellini beans)
- 1 small carrot, peeled and cubed
- 1 celery stalk, diced
- ½ small onion, peeled and chopped
- 1 clove of garlic, chopped
- 2 cups spring water
- 1 tsp extra virgin olive oil
- ¼ tsp dried thyme
- ¼ tsp dried oregano
- ½ tsp parsley or dill (for garnish)

### Instructions:

1. Heat olive oil to medium heat and sauté chopped garlic in a small pot. Add spring water and white beans and let it cook for 1 hour.
2. add chopped onion, cubed carrot, and celery stalk after the white beans and cook for 20-30 minutes. Add thyme, oregano, and black pepper. Mix well.
3. Transfer in a bowl and garnish with fresh parsley or dill.
4. Serve immediately.

Total calories: 216   Carbohydrates: 32g
Proteins: 8.6g      Fat: 5g

## 6. Cashew Hummus and Veggie Sandwich

Prep Time: 10 minutes| Chill Time: 4 hrs| Total Time: 4 hrs 10 mins| Difficulty: Easy

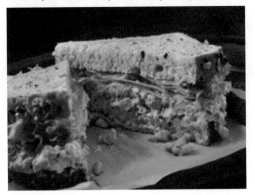

### Ingredients:

- For the cashew hummus:
- ½ cup cashews, soaked overnight
- ½ clove of garlic
- 1 tsp lime juice
- 1 tsp extra virgin olive oil
- 1/8 tsp cumin powder
- 1/8 tsp black pepper
- 2-4 drops of water (to adjust the consistency)
-
- For the Veggie Sandwich:
- two slices of whole wheat sourdough bread
- ¼ avocado, sliced
- ½ cucumber sliced
- ½ cup lettuce leaves

### Instructions:

1. For the cashew hummus, blend the soaked cashews and the other ingredients in a food processor or blender until smooth and creamy.
2. Now, take a whole wheat sourdough bread slice and spread cashew hummus over it. Layer sliced avocado, cucumber, and lettuce leaves over it and make a sandwich.
3. Serve immediately.

Total calories: 646  Carbohydrates: 53.8g      Proteins: 17g      Fat: 41.6g

## 7. Black Bean and Lime-infused Corn Salad

Prep Time: 10 minutes| Chill Time: 4 hrs| Total Time: 4 hrs 10 mins| Difficulty: Easy

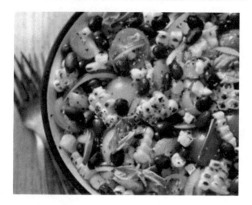

### Ingredients:

- ½ cup canned black beans, choose low sodium drained and rinsed well
- ½ cup fresh or canned corn kernels drained and rinsed well
- ¼ avocado sliced
- ¼ cup cherry tomatoes, chopped
- ½ small onion, peeled and chopped
- Few fresh cilantro leaves
- 1 tsp lime juice
- 1/8 tsp black pepper
- Pinch of cayenne pepper for a spicy kick

### Instructions:

1. Combine all the ingredients in a bowl.
2. Mix it well.
3. Serve immediately.

## 8. Mango & Pineapple Yogurt Parfait

Prep Time: 10 minutes| Chill Time: 30 mins| Total Time: 40 mins| Difficulty: Easy

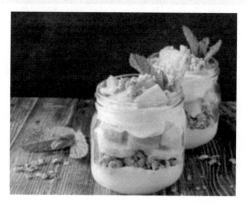

### Ingredients:

- ½ cup almond yogurt
- ½ cup mango chunks
- ½ cup pineapple chunks
- 2 tbsp granola
- 5g walnuts, crushed

### Instructions:

1. Add ¼ cups of almond yogurt to a jar. Add a layer of half granola, followed by ¼ cup of mango and pineapple chunks.
2. Repeat the layers. Refrigerate it for 30 minutes before serving.
3. Top it with crushed walnuts and enjoy.

Total calories: 292  Carbohydrates: 46.6g  Proteins: 11.2g  Fat: 9.1g

Total calories: 273  Carbohydrates: 48.7g  Proteins: 4.7g  Fat: 10.5g

## 1. Mixed Berries White Bean Smoothie

Prep Time: 10 minutes| Cook Time: 0 mins|
Total Time: 10 mins| Difficulty: Easy

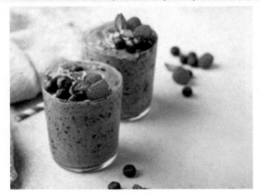

### Ingredients:

- 1 cup fresh or frozen mixed berries
- ½ cup cooked white beans (preferably navy or cannellini)
- ½ cup almond milk
- ¼ cup almond yogurt
- 1 tsp acacia honey
- 1 tsp flax seeds
- Ice cubes as needed

### Instructions:

1. Place all the ingredients in a blender and blend on high speed until you achieve a smooth and creamy consistency.
2. If the smoothie is too thick, add half a cup of almond milk to adjust the consistency.
3. Transfer the smoothie into a glass and garnish with mixed berries.

Total calories: 258  Carbohydrates: 42g
Proteins: 10g      Fat: 6.5g

## 2. Red Cabbage, Carrot & Cucumber Coleslaw

Prep Time: 15 minutes| Cook Time: 0 mins|
Total Time: 15 mins| Difficulty: Easy

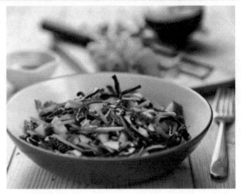

### Ingredients:

- ½ cup red cabbage, sliced
- one small carrot, peeled and julienned cut
- one small cucumber cubed
- For dressing:
- 1 tsp rice vinegar
- ½ tsp mustard seeds
- 1 tsp cilantro leaves
- Sea salt and black pepper as per taste

### Instructions:

1. Combine all the vegetables in a bowl.
2. Prepare the dressing by mixing rice vinegar, salt, black pepper, and cilantro leaves.
3. Sprinkle mustard seeds on top and serve.

Total calories: 150 Carbohydrates:
20gProteins: 2g      Fat: 2g

### 3. Green Kale Salad with Cranberries and Avocado

Prep Time: 15 minutes| Cook time: 0 mins| Total Time: 15 mins| Difficulty: Easy

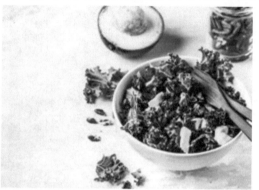

**Ingredients:**

- 1 cup fresh kale leaves, chopped
- ¼ avocado, pitted and cubed
- ½ cup dried cranberries
- 1 tsp lemon juice
- one tsp extra virgin olive oil
- 1 tsp pumpkin seeds (optional)
- 5g walnuts
- Sea salt and black pepper as per taste

**Instructions:**

1. Combine all the ingredients in a bowl.
2. Sprinkle pumpkin seeds and crushed walnuts on top.
3. Serve immediately.

Total calories: 628  Carbohydrates: 65g
Proteins: 7g      Fat:14g

### 4. Three Bean Salad

Prep Time: 15 minutes| Cook time: 0 mins| Total Time: 15 mins| Difficulty: Easy

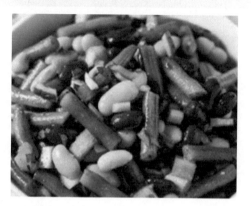

**Ingredients:**

- ½ cup green beans
- ½ cup canned red kidney beans drained and rinsed well
- ½ cup white beans (preferably cannellini)
- Few fresh cilantro leaves
- 1 tsp apple cider vinegar
- 1 tsp extra virgin olive oil
- 1/8 tsp paprika powder
- 1/8 tsp garlic powder
- ¼ tsp. garlic powder

**Instructions:**

1. Combine all the ingredients in a bowl, toss well.
2. Add paprika powder, garlic powder, black pepper, lime juice, and apple cider vinegar to the salad. Mix well.
3. Sprinkle cilantro leaves on top and enjoy.

Total calories: 318 Carbohydrates: 49.8g  Proteins: 18g      Fat: 5g

## 5. Raw Spinach & Avocado Smoothie

Prep Time: 10 minutes| Cook time: 0 mins|
Total Time: 15 mins| Difficulty: Easy

## 6. Raw Broccoli & Peanut Salad

Prep Time: 10 minutes| Cook Time: 0 mins|
Total Time: 15 mins| Difficulty: Easy

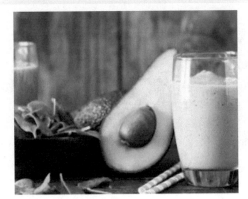

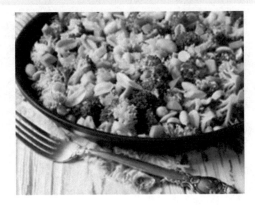

### Ingredients:

- 1 cup fresh baby spinach leaves
- ½ avocado, pitted and sliced
- ½ cup almond milk or any plant-based milk of your choice
- ½ small banana
- ¼ cup almond yogurt
- 1 tsp chia seeds
- 1 tsp avocado honey
- Ice cubes as needed

### Instructions:

1. Blend all ingredients at high speed until you achieve a smooth & creamy consistency.
2. If the smoothie is too thick, add half a cup of almond milk to get the desired consistency.
3. Serve immediately.

### Ingredients:

- ½ cup broccoli florets
- 1 small carrot, peeled and cubed
- 2 tbsp peanuts
- 1 tsp lime juice
- 1 tsp apple cider vinegar

### Instructions:

1. Combine broccoli florets, cubed carrot, lime juice, and apple cider vinegar in a bowl. Mix well.
2. Sprinkle peanuts on the top of salad.
3. Serve immediately.

Total calories: 261  Carbohydrates: 31.4g
Proteins: 5.6g     Fat: 15.5g

Total calories: 135    Carbohydrates: 12.8g    Proteins: 6.7g    Fat: 8.4g

## 7. Roasted sweet potato with rosemary

Prep Time: 5 minutes| Cook Time: 20mins| Total Time: 15 mins| Difficulty: Easy

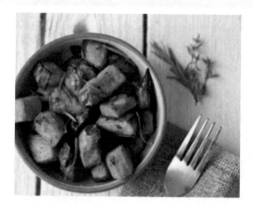

**Ingredients:**

- 1 medium sweet potato
- 1 tsp olive oil
- 1 tsp fresh rosemary, chopped
- ¼ tsp garlic powder

**Instructions:**

1. Preheat oven to 200 C for 5-10 minutes.
2. Cut sweet potato into equal cubes.
3. Grease the baking tray with olive oil and spread the sweet potato cubes over the tray.
4. Roast them for 20 minutes until a golden-brown color is achieved.
5. Garnish fresh rosemary leaves on the top.
6. Serve immediately.

Total calories: 157   Carbohydrates: 27.1g   Proteins: 2.2g   Fat: 4.7g

## 8. Raw Lettuce & Peach Salad

Prep Time: 10 minutes| Cook Time: 0 mins| Total Time: 15 mins| Difficulty: Easy

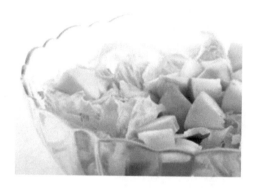

**Ingredients:**

- ½ cup lettuce leaves
- ½ cup spinach leaves
- one small peach, sliced
- ¼ cup feta cheese
- 5g crushed pecans

**Instructions:**

1. Combine all ingredients except the pecans in a bowl.
2. Top it with crushed pecans.
3. Serve immediately.

Total calories: 185   Carbohydrates: 19g   Proteins: 6g   Fat: 10g

# 1. Flax seed energy balls

Prep Time: 10 minutes| Cook Time: 0 mins|
Total Time: 15 mins|  Difficulty: Easy

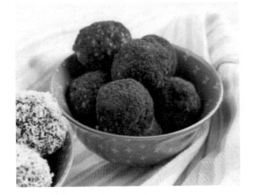

**Ingredients:**

- 4 tbsp cup flax seeds
- 4 tbsp rolled oats
- 1 tbsp sunflower seeds
- 1 tbsp pumpkin seeds
- 2 tbsp dried figs, chopped
- 2 tbsp raw honey
- 1 tsp coconut oil
- Pinch of cinnamon powder
- ¼ tsp vanilla extract
- 1 tbsp shredded coconut

**Instructions:**

1. Roast all the seeds in a saucepan for 2-3 minutes.
2. Slightly heat honey, coconut oil, and vanilla extract for 1 minute in a separate pan.
3. Combine the wet and dry ingredients.
4. Using your hands, roll this mixture into a ball shape.
5. Serve immediately.

# 2. Turmeric & Lime Roasted Chickpeas

Prep Time: 10 minutes| Cook Time: 25mins|
Total Time: 35 mins|  Difficulty: Easy

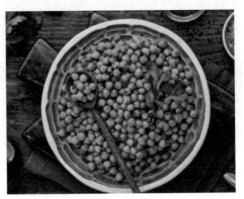

**Ingredients:**

- One can 15-ounce chickpeas
- 1 tbsp olive oil
- Juice of 1 lime
- 1/8 tsp turmeric powder
- 1/8 tsp Sea salt
- 1/8 tsp paprika powder

**Instructions:**

1. Preheat your oven to 200 C.
2. In a medium bowl, add the drained chickpeas, turmeric powder, sea salt, and paprika powder. Mix well until the chickpeas are coated evenly.
3. Place the coated chickpeas in a baking tray greased with olive oil and roast for 20-25 minutes until golden brown.
4. After the chickpeas are roasted, squeeze the juice of one lemon over them.
5. Serve them warm.

Total calories: 683 Carbohydrates: 81g    Proteins: 13g    Fat: 27.8g

Total calories: 471 Carbohydrates: 57g    Proteins: 18g    Fat: 21g

## 3. Creamy Strawberry & Banana Smoothie

Prep Time: 10 minutes| Cook Time: 0 mins|
Total Time: 10 mins| Difficulty: Easy

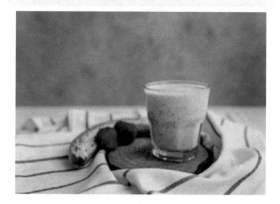

## 4. Apple & Cinnamon Chips

Prep Time: 10 minutes| Cook Time: 0 mins|
Total Time: 15 mins| Difficulty: Easy

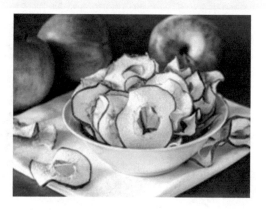

### Ingredients:

- ½ cup fresh or frozen strawberries
- ½ small banana
- ½ cup almond milk
- 1 tbsp oats
- 1 tbsp chia seeds
- 1 tbsp raw honey
- Pinch of cinnamon powder
- Ice cubes as needed

### Instructions:

1. Blend all ingredients on high speed until you achieve a smooth & creamy consistency.
2. Transfer this smoothie into a glass & garnish with some strawberries.
3. Serve immediately.

### Ingredients:

- one large apple
- ¼ tsp cinnamon powder
- 1 tsp manuka honey

### Instructions:

1. Preheat oven to 110 C for 5-10 minutes.
2. Cut the apple into thin round rings. Place them on a baking tray and sprinkle cinnamon powder and manuka honey on top.
3. Bake them for 1-1.5 hours until they get crunchy and crispy.
4. Transfer them to a serving plate & serve.

Total calories: 253 Carbohydrates: 48.9g   Proteins: 5.4g     Fat: 6.3g

Total calories: 471 Carbohydrates: 57g   Proteins: 18g     Fat: 21g

## 5. Dried Figs Energy Bars

Prep Time: 10 minutes| Cook Time: 0 mins|
Total Time: 40 mins| Difficulty: Easy

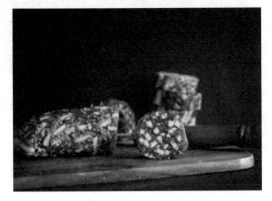

### Ingredients:

- Five dried figs
- 2 tbsp oats
- 1 tbsp sesame seeds
- 1 tbsp pumpkin seeds
- 1 tbsp raw honey
- 1 tbsp coconut oil
- Pinch of cinnamon

### Instructions:

1. Combine all the dry and wet ingredients until they combine well.
2. Place this mixture on a tray, press it firmly, and cut the bars into a rectangular shape.
3. Refrigerate for 30 minutes until they achieve a more combined texture.

Total calories: 454 Carbohydrates: 57.8g   Proteins: 7.7g   Fat: 20.3g

## 6. Sweet Honey & Paprika Seasoned Corn

Prep Time: 10 minutes| Cook Time: 0 mins|
Total Time: 15 mins| Difficulty: Easy

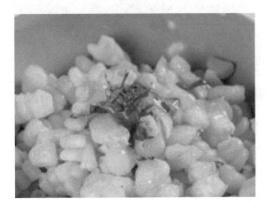

### Ingredients:

- ½ cup canned corn, boiled
- 1 tsp honey
- 1/8 tsp paprika powder

### Instructions:

1. Combine corn, honey, and paprika powder in a bowl. Mix it well.
2. Serve immediately.

Total calories: 82 Carbohydrates: 20g
Proteins: 2.1g   Fat: 1g

## 7. Cinnamon Infused French Toast

Prep Time: 5 minutes| Cook Time: 10 mins| Total Time: 15 mins| Difficulty: Easy

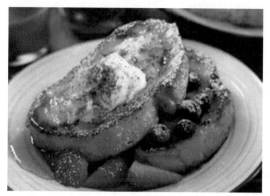

### Ingredients:

- one medium egg, beaten
- 1 tbsp honey
- 1 tbsp extra virgin olive oil
- two whole wheat bread slices
- 1 tsp sesame seeds
- 1 sliced banana

### Instructions:

1. Mix the beaten egg, honey, sesame seeds, and cinnamon powder in a bowl.
2. Heat olive oil in a nonstick pan.
3. Now dip the bread slice in this egg mixture, put it in the pan, and toast it for 2-3 minutes on each side until it turns golden brown.
4. Garnish with sliced banana and drizzle a layer of honey on top.

## 8. Pineapple & Granola Yogurt Parfait Bowl

Prep Time: 10 minutes| Cook Time: 0 mins| Total Time: 15 mins| Difficulty: Easy

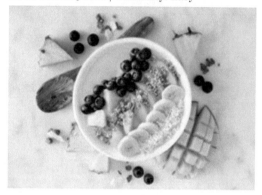

### Ingredients:

- ½ cup coconut yogurt
- 2 tbsp granola
- 1 tbsp shredded coconut
- ½ cup fresh pineapple chunks

### Instructions:

1. Add ¼ cup of coconut yogurt to a jar, followed by half a cup of granola and ¼ cup of pineapple chunks.
2. Repeat the layers.
3. Garnish it with shredded coconut on top.
4. Refrigerate it for 30 minutes before serving.

Total calories: 444  Carbohydrates: 43.6g   Proteins: 13,7g    Fat: 25.5g

Total calories: 244  Carbohydrates: 30.5gProteins: 3.9g    Fat: 14.6g

# ALLERGEN-SAFE COOKING: HELPFUL TIPS AND TRICKS

The Food Allergen Labelling and Consumer Protection Act of 2004 (FALCPA) lists soybeans, milk, eggs, fish, tree nuts, crustacean shellfish, peanuts, and wheat as significant allergens.

The FDA enforces FALCPA compliance in food labeling, except for poultry, meats, egg products, and most alcoholic drinks, which are regulated by other Federal authorities. FALCPA standards require product labels to prominently identify food source names if an ingredient corresponds to one of the eight identified food allergies or includes protein from one of these foods. Reading labels may help food allergy sufferers avoid certain foods.

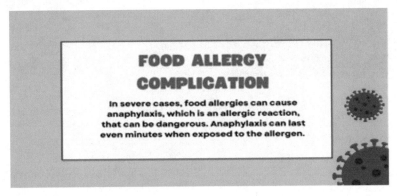

## Identification of allergens on food labels

Food labels should mention food allergens like:

Parenthesis after ingredient names in ingredient list. Example: "Lecithin (Soy)", "Flour (wheat)" and "Whey (Milk)"

A "contain" remark after or adjacent to the components. Example: "Contains" Wheat, Milk or Soy.

# Substitutes for Allergen Ingredients

No one's favorite foods should be automatically off-limits to those with food allergies. If an allergen is present, various alternatives may be used in its place. Below are a few other options for allergenic foods that are often unavailable.

**Milk:** Studies have shown that soy milk is the healthiest choice because it contains about the same amount of protein, vitamin D, and calcium as conventional milk. Almond, rice, and cashew milk also provide about the same amount of calcium and vitamin D, but they're low in fat and protein.

**Eggs:** If you are allergic to eggs, you may easily replace them in many recipes with apple sauce, flaxseed, or pureed bananas. These substitutes play essential roles, such as binding, moisturizing, and leavening, to ensure that allergen-free meals remain flavorful.

**Fish:** Meals that include fish may be prepared using plant-based food or other non-fish protein alternatives for those allergic to fish. Tempeh or tofu has high protein content and adaptability; you can spice those soy-based alternatives to taste and feel like fish. The flaky texture of jackfruit is also reminiscent of fish. Because of their meaty texture, mushrooms (such as Shiitake) may be cooked and seasoned in various ways to make them taste like fish.

**Peanuts:** A popular peanut-free substitute, sunflower seed butter has a comparable creamy texture and is versatile enough to be used in baking, sauces, and spreads. Almond butter is also an excellent substitute for peanut butter, but it won't work for those allergic to tree nuts.

**Wheat:** Almond flour is a great gluten-free and low-carb substitute. It adds a nutty taste and a moist texture to baked goods and meals. Rice flour is also a gluten-free option with a neutral taste. It can be used to create noodles, thicken sauces, and bake.

# Strategies to Prevent Allergen Exposure in Kitchen

**Storage Area:** Store allergen-free goods in designated containers with clear labels to avoid cross-contamination.

**Utensils:** For allergen-safe food prep, keep utensils, cutting boards, and cookware separate.
Labeling: Mark all food items, storage containers, and areas. Clearly labeling everything helps families with various food allergies or intolerances stay safe.

**Cleaning:** Use soapy, hot water to wash surfaces, dishes, and appliances regularly

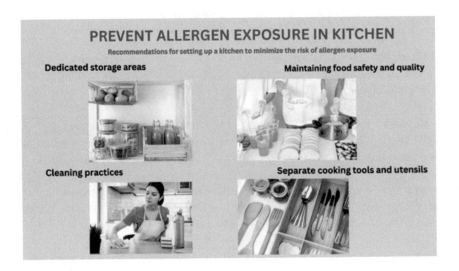

## Collaboration with Healthcare Specialists

To properly accommodate particular allergies, it is essential to collaborate with healthcare specialists in creating anti-inflammatory diets. Collaboration between nutritionists, allergists, and dietitians may lead to developing individualized eating programs that mitigate allergic reactions by lowering inflammation. By working closely with these professionals, you can ensure your diet is healthy and provides all the nutrients you need. In addition to advising on safe replacements for allergies like wheat, nuts, and dairy, healthcare professionals may help choose foods that reduce inflammation, like spices, fatty fish substitutes (such as walnuts and chis seeds), and leafy greens. Ensuring that the diet is both health-promoting and allergen-free, regular follow-ups and changes further boost its efficacy. By working together, we can help people take charge of their health and give them the confidence they need to eat well without worrying about side effects.

# CHAPTER 5

## Meal Planning and Advanced Prep Techniques

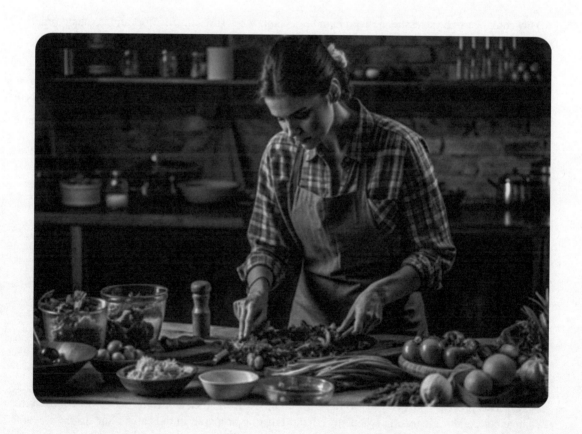

Advanced preparation techniques can be very handy for efficient meal planning. The following are some practical tips for advanced meal preparation that can easily be incorporated into daily life.

# Batch Cooking for the Week Ahead

Planning and cooking daily can be cumbersome and exhaustive. It involves a significant amount of time deciding what to buy, where to buy from, and cooking every meal from scratch. Batch cooking techniques help overcome these issues associated with daily planning and cooking. It allows bulk shopping at a cheaper price and saves cooking time, energy, and resources. A well-balanced diet is adequate and proportionate in terms of nutrients. Ensuring the inclusion of all food groups in the right amount daily becomes a real challenge. Batch cooking for a week helps to plan nutritionally adequate diets for the longer term. For instance, a missed animal protein source at one time can be compensated at another mealtime. Similarly, a planned dine-out (which may be high in sodium or fat) can be compensated for with low sodium or less fatty food the next day.

Daily cooking can be stressful. A menu plan for a whole week saves much effort and is a good practice for organizing meals.
Following is the step-by-step guide for batch cooking:

- Select a day you will plan for the whole week. This day can be chosen based on your daily schedule or your family's routine. Sunday is a good day for many people.
- Choose a suitable time of day for planning. Schedule a minimum of 30 minutes for the task.
- Take an inventory of the stored food items at home.
- Write down the names of seven dishes according t the family's choice and your resources.
- Arrange the meal items according to their similarity of ingredients into days of the week on which they would be served

After deciding what to cook each day, it is helpful to cook similar ingredients and store them according to the suitable preservation method. For instance, if you plan to use chicken stock in two recipes on two different days, you may prepare the bulk of stock at a single time and freeze the rest. However, always preserve the food in usable bits (according to single-time usage in separate storage boxes). This prevents the necessity to thaw the complete food stock and refreeze it. Some food items change color, odor, or texture when stored and must be prepared immediately. For instance, when cooled, some sauces change their texture, which cannot be returned to normal. In this case, you might need to ensure that the sauce ingredients are fully prepared but not thickened.

### Efficient Use of Freezer Meals

Freezing is an efficient method of food preservation. We usually use freezing to keep individual ingredients, but it can also efficiently store cooked meals for quick use. For this purpose, storage boxes to contain a one-time usage portion of a meal can be very handy. The storage boxes can be labeled with the name and date of freezing simply by using masking tape and pen. This helps to quickly locate food items without thawing. The boxes can be stored in the usage sequence (Friday food items are to be stored at the back while Monday ones are to be stored in front).

Additionally, old stock of food items can be rotated after each week so that they are utilized in next week's menu before expiry. Several foods, including ready-to-fry, cook, heat, or serve items, can be frozen depending upon the weekly meal plan. Diced vegetables, stir-fried vegetables, cooked spinach, boiled or marinated meat, ready-to-fry burger patties, soups without thickening agents, boiled beans, and to-heat gravies are some of the items you can quickly refrigerate for one day or store in freezer for a longer time as per need

### Spice Mixes and Marinades to Prep in Advance

Certain spices or base recipes are used in several dishes depending on the cuisine. Stored spice mixes (especially in powdered form) are quite helpful for long-term usage. Quick mixes of recipes are available, too. Some marinades and sauces (the most common of which is tomato paste) can also be frozen for future usage. In addition to the flavor, marinades can provide additional benefits such as ease of preparation and health. Marinades containing garlic paste can add to the anti-inflammatory properties. Cooked or uncooked tomato paste containing blended garlic, ginger, and onion can be used in several gravies and as a general thickening agent. Sauces and marinades may include an assortment of spices that have health benefits, including anti-inflammatory properties, such as turmeric, mixed herbs, anise, cardamom, cinnamon, and fennel seeds. Cinnamon powder is beneficial for adding quick flavor to recipes as simple as French toast. The mint paste can be made and stored in the refrigerator for a week for yogurt or sandwiches.

### Themed Meal Nights to Simplify Planning

Involving family members in menu planning can create inclusivity and strengthen the relationship and bond. "Theme meal nights" such as Meatless Day, No Sugar Day, Vegetarian Day, or "Cuisine meal nights" such as South Asian, Italian, Chinese, etc. can make meal planning a happy family time. All family members can be involved by allocating one day to each family member, for example, Sam's Monday, Andy's Tuesday, etc. The person might be responsible for giving meal ideas and/or cooking the meals as per the age or skill of the family member. The rules/aims must be kept in mind while planning the meals. For instance, "Anti Inflammatory Week" can include recipes containing herbs, spices, nuts, and other plant-based foods with known antioxidant and anti-inflammatory properties.

## Using Leftovers Wisely to Minimize Waste

Weekly menu planning helps reduce daily food waste. There can be some recipes that utilize similar ingredients. Upon properly planning the week's menu, these recipes can be kept on consecutive days to reduce food waste. Similarly, there must be flexibility in menu planning to incorporate any change in case of unexpected food wastage. Some ideas for effective utilization of leftovers include using a leftover steak in a sandwich for the next day, using leftover rice in rice balls/snacks, putting the leftover gravy in steamed rice, mixing leftover beans with boiled potatoes to form cutlets, etc. Leftovers can even be blended and used to form crepes. There are people in the world who don't have food to eat. Ethical and economic reasons exist for using leftover foods with much care and planning. However, caution must be exerted while handling leftovers. They must not be refrozen, for example, to prevent food-borne illnesses.

## Seasonal Meal Planning for Freshness and Economy

Seasonal foods (fruits and vegetables) are cheaper than imported or out-of-season items. Weekly menu plans must involve seasonal items for the sake of economy, freshness, and nutrition. Out-of-season foods are obviously not fresh, and if they are, they may have been preserved in some way. Some nutrients, such as Vitamin C, are very sensitive and start disappearing from fruit as early as it is harvested. You have a very good option of enjoying fresh and nutritious food at a cheaper rate if you choose seasonal items. For the best seasonal options, a farmer's market is a better bet than the average grocery store.

Here are some tips for identifying seasonal items:

- The food items available in large stocks at cheap rates
- Google the food's harvesting cycle
- Go for local produce, explore what your area is known for producing
- Go to a fresh stock market (suburban markets, weekend markets)

Some internet trends urge people to buy food items that are mentioned on social media. Though this practice is okay for occasional use, it can incur high economic and even health costs in the long run. You may always find local alternatives for foods available in the market. This helps to support the local farmers, too. Here are some examples of other options that you may use in your meal planning:

- Healthy fats rich foods (Fatty fish/ walnuts/ cashews/ almonds/ pumpkin seeds/ flax seeds/ chia seeds)

- Antioxidant-rich foods (Choose a variety of colored foods available in the market, such as red, yellow, orange, green, and purple fruits and vegetables)

Foods are grouped in food groups according to their similar active ingredients. Specific foods are not necessary; a variety of options are available with similar nutrient profiles while maintaining local, seasonal items. A well-planned weekly menu ensures that all nutritional requirements are fulfilled while decreasing workload and costs.

# CHAPTER 6

## *Overcoming Challenges and Staying Motivated*

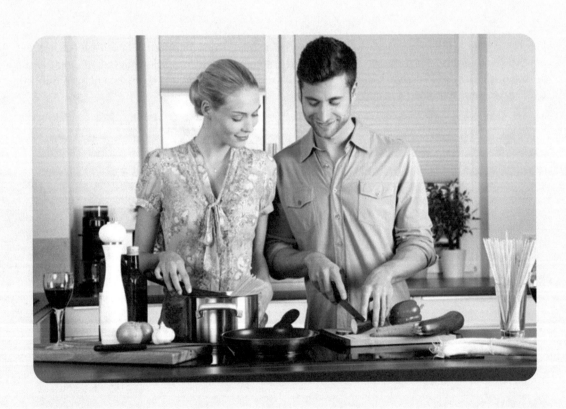

Meal planning and preparation can be challenging in terms of the effort required. On busy days, it is very important to read tips on how to manage time, money, and motivation around cooking and eating. The following are some tips that will keep you motivated to overcome the challenges of meal preparation.

## Overcoming the Time Barrier: Quick Tips for Faster Prep

In this era, time is the most significant property that one possesses. Any tip to organize an efficient work routine is a lifesaver. It can prevent long-term burnout and give a sense of achievement upon completing the task.

Meal preparation using multipurpose and ready-to-use items such as multipurpose flour, self-raising flour, instant yeast, pre-roasted cereals, frozen stir-fried vegetables, precook mixes, spice mixes, and sauces. These cooking ingredients can be home-prepared for a week's or month's usage and stored for long-term usage.

Cooking sessions can be organized based on relevant tasks such as dicing vegetables for two days and stored in the freezer, marinating meats for two days at a time, grocery shopping for the whole week, and keeping the most commonly used ready-to-cook mixes in stock.

Such practices help save time around starting each batch of cooking from scratch and also cater to emergencies such as power outages or unexpected guests. Sometimes, cutting vegetables can be much of a task in recipes, and if that part is already done, mixing, making a sauce, or seasoning does not remain much of a task. For example, Chinese food recipes require a lot of time cutting vegetables.

Salads and fruit mixes follow a similar pattern. Cutting all meals throughout the day into small chunks increases the time required for preparation, like washing a cutting board, preparing a knife, washing, peeling, and cutting each food, closing the whole process, and then doing it again in a small chunk for the following recipe.

It is an excellent organizing technique to arrange similar tasks simultaneously because it requires less mental burden. Pre-cut and pre-washed options of various foods, including vegetables and meats, are also available but usually at a higher price.

Only you can decide if saving time if worth the cost. Maintaining a balance between cost and convenience is necessary, and this choice varies.

Pressure cooking, microwave cooking, and air frying help cook food faster and/or healthier than their counterparts. Such technology is highly useful if convenience is sought. Air fryers save a lot of oil, which is economical and nutritious. Pressure cooking saves a lot of time, especially while tenderizing tough cuts of meat. Available technologies must be used in the best possible way to avoid excessive fatigue or a toll on health.

## Eating Well on a Tight Budget

In industrialized societies, fresh foods come at a higher price than processed or ready-to-eat foods. It is generally believed that eating healthy is always heavy on the wallet. However, proper meal planning can provide budget-friendly alternatives to costly items. Eating local and seasonal is the key. One great option for purchasing budget-friendly foods is farmer markets. You may choose local varieties of fish, nuts, seeds, fruits, and vegetables to keep your budget low and select healthy options. Well-fed industrialized societies usually post what we see online, and people think it is the only option available. However, the tip is to buy whatever fresh produce is available in your market and just go for it. If avocados are unavailable, go for olives; if chia seeds are unavailable, go for flax seeds; if citrus fruits are unavailable, go for guavas.

Some foods, such as Greek Yogurt or Cottage Cheese, are expensive when bought from stores but can be made at home. Even bread, simple yogurt, and spice mixes can be made at home. Highly convenient foods such as fried onions are available on the market. You can buy those if you prioritize time and convenience. However, you must decide if you can invest some of your time to make such products at home and save money. The long-term investment in health by using better quality oil to fry those onions must also be considered while making choices. In other words, healthier foods are budget-friendly but come with a bit of inconvenience. You must balance your daily routine, delegate tasks, use machines to reduce workload, and save time by bulk buying and preparing.

## Dealing with Dietary Burnout: Keeping Meals Interesting

As described in the previous chapter, weekly meal planning allows for cuisine-based planning and ensures dietary diversity.

- Monotonous meal patterns are not healthy for physical as well as for mental health.
- Mealtimes should be fun; family members will get together at a feast they find interesting.
- A weekly menu plan allows for dealing with burnout and provides a fresh start with similar yet different recipes throughout all days.
- Besides cuisine-themed menus, you may go for seasonal menus such as soups, which are more commonly consumed in winter, and fresh fruit juices, etc., in summer.
- Similarly, fresh fruits and vegetables in season automatically add to a variety in the diet. Such a variation allows for the cherishing of change with motivation and passion.
- Follow social media pages with tips on swapping food ingredients for palatability, change, and discover innovative food preparation ideas.
- Try new cuisines and cultural recipes, and exchange ideas at social gatherings to keep things interesting in a dull life.
- More minds can be involved in menu planning.
- They can all come together to offer something new rather than a monotonous routine.
- Keep a record of the old week's menu and repeat the menus with alternative swapping of individual courses on meals served in the first week per se.
- Even small changes, such as garnishing, can freshen everyone's mind and mood at the table.

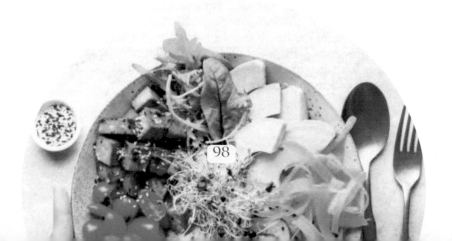

# Social Eating: Sticking to Your Diet at Parties and Restaurants

Social eating can be kept a part of the weekly menu, but if an unexpected birthday party comes up, what will you do? No worries, just adjust some of the eating patterns to match a part of the week's menu to a maximum extent.

You may alternate the portion of planned fish with a lean steak or chicken if fish is unavailable on the party menu. But don't go way beyond what you intended. Even if something unplanned is very appetizing or exciting, you must go for it only for a small portion. You can adjust the weekly menu the next day according to what you eat at the party.

You may even have a small meal before social gatherings or grocery shopping to avoid unintentionally eating large portions of unhealthy items for the sake of hunger.

One dish party offers a variety of options without compromising your meal pattern. You may choose to make a main dish on your menu for all people at a party and choose a similar second course on your menu that is available at the party.

Make healthy eating a positive discussion at the party so that other people also become educated to make healthy, homemade, safe food options.

You may choose to set a trend of, for example, "no carbonated beverage party," or bring something useful or healthy to the host's house, such as milk packages rather than a bakery item.

## Building a Support Network for Diet Success

Intrinsic motivation is a great quality to have. But sometimes you need extrinsic motivation to keep moving during the lows. A supportive community helps you to successfully follow your planned diet. A "partner in healthy meals" will be effective in longer term commitment. If one gets demotivated, the other one supports and levels things up. It gives a sense of accountability through external pressure which is frequently needed at some point in life. Social media talks, public and private groups are quite useful for finding similar minded people. Networking also helps in exchanging ideas and tips and to read motivational success stories. Partnering in the meal buying, preparing and cooking helps in division of work and introduces a sense of long-term commitment by preventing burnout. You may always sit together or have an online meetup with your 'anti-inflammatory diet partner' and talk about your previous week's successes and points of improvements.

# Tracking Progress: Tools and Tips for Seeing Results

The whole purpose of weekly planning is to delay gratification, Instant results usually come with a price and make a person stuck in daily grind.

On the other hand, long term plans allow room for flexibility and are more efficient. But being realistic about goals while setting weekly plans is very important.

You must not be overly rigid about healthy meals. The goal that it compromises your time and effort and failure demotivates you for your next days.

Each day should be flexible yet planned. If it is someone's birthday, enjoy a small piece of cake and watch your eating habits for the rest of the week.

Keeping records on mobile apps with daily reminders can help long term storage of data rather than using pen and diary. Finding an old menu is easy to do in digital format.

You may upload and save the comments/ pictures or family members on each day so that you can improve the menu for the next time or remember what was the tastiest items at the previous get-together.

You may choose to keep a long-term health goal such as reducing free sugar intake.

You may start with a small deduction of obvious sugar sources going forward toward reducing sweetened beverages, sweets, snacks and desserts etc.

You may keep a record of how well you have come through the whole process of reducing sugar in your diet. Goals are achieved one small step at a time.

One less cookie a at a time. It motivates and helps you keep a sense of self efficacy.

You may decide on a monthly date on which you target to renew or take the next stride in changing a dietary choice. A small notch up in reducing sugar in coffee, for example, can help you slowly develop taste.

Quick fixes and bulky changes are usually short term and associated with a big setback. Slow and steady wins the health!

# CHAPTER 7

*Beyond the Diet: Lifestyle Integration*

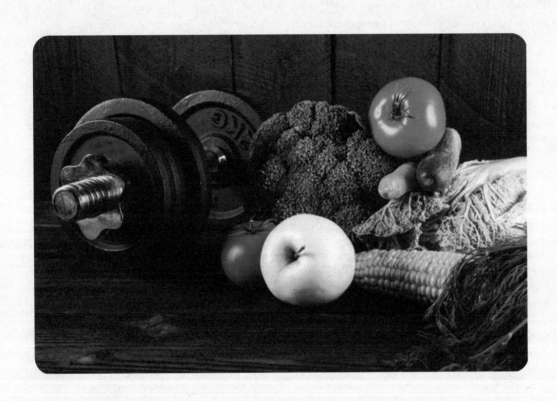

Diet alone is not a game changer. You need to have an overall healthy lifestyle including exercise, sleep patterns, stress reduction and complementary therapies for reducing the inflammation.

# Anti-Inflammatory Exercise Routines

Regular physical activity is linked to a healthier mental and physical self. Inflammation may result in joint, bone and muscle pains and fatigue.

But if you reduce your activity pattern, it only worsens the condition. When you move your body against gravity, the muscles, bones and joints get stronger. This is why bedridden patients lose calcium from their bones and lose strength in muscles.

Blood circulation increases when your muscles demand more oxygen and glucose because of movement. This blood takes away the toxins produced in muscles and clears away the waste materials.

However, you don't need to be athletic on one hand and completely sedentary on the other. There is a way in between which is sustainable for a longer time.

You may choose the sports of your interest including swimming, cycling, tennis, badminton or go for a yoga class. One hour of physical activity routine per day has known benefits for mental and physical health.

You may split your exercise routine into parts such as 15 minutes of walking before breakfast, 30 minutes of outdoor sports, and 15 minutes of yoga in the evening. Sustainability is the key.

You must not target a one-hour gym session on the first day and start off with heavy weight lifting. You need to acclimate your body slowly to engage in one more set of exercises each day. Keep it all happy too. Otherwise, you might lose interest.

An exercise partner is a good way of linking social life with exercise. In daily life, you need to find out ways to alternate sedentary pattern with active patterns such as parking the car a bit far away from your office building to walk through that path, use stairs instead of elevator for at least one time a day, take breaks during work, explore office chair exercises including stretching and breathing, put reminder of phone to take a break after every 40-60 minutes.

We need to reduce our sitting time throughout the day through simple ways which are easy to integrate into daily practice.

## Stress Reduction Techniques That Complement Your Diet

Chronic inflammation is associated with several non-communicable diseases such as bone and joint diseases, diabetes, and cardiovascular problems.

It can be exacerbated by stress.

Therefore, reducing and managing stress is essential for maintaining a healthy lifestyle. Mindfulness practices, yoga and breathing exercises help in reducing stress and can have an impact on inflammatory markers.

There are mobile apps available for this purpose, as well, which have self-paced courses on guided meditation.

In addition, physical activity can have huge mental health benefits.

A simple walk in the garden, seeing colors, taking breaks, painting or doing art activity, aromatherapy help in relieving stress with the least amount of time investment.

Be sure to include routine breaks from work and enjoying some work free days.

The Internet and mobile phones can be quite stressful too.

You might decide to have a no internet day for example to cut yourself off and spend time with nature or family.

Everyone has their own triggers to stress. You need to identify your trigger, what makes you feel as you do, and work on ways to deal with the situation.

Having knowledge about how you feel using the emotion wheel or other aids of psychology helps to identify and then resolve a problem.

You may keep a record of your physical symptoms of stress including heavy breathing, high blood pressure, headache, disturbed sleep, and try to identify what happened before it occurred.

These identified predecessors will help you resolve the issues through talking or assertive communication with others. Safe connections are highly beneficial in stress management.

## Sleep Optimization for Better Health

Sleep is a big factor involved in stress management. If you are sleep deprived, you will get easily irritated and fatigued. On the other hand, if you are stressed out, your sleep pattern may get disturbed. Eight hours of sleep per day is a must.

You might need to take necessary actions to help yourself get to sleep in an optimum fashion. These include purging yourself from any light before sleeping. Mobile or LED lights hinder sleep and keep you awake.

You need to signal your body that the sun is down and it is time to sleep. Light pollution makes your body receptors confused and affects your body clock in a negative way. So, reading a book in hard copy is a better way of bedtime routine.

You may choose to apply certain soothing oils/masks or other relaxation techniques to help your body prepare for sleep time. Similarly, natural sleeping agents such as primrose oil, herbal tea, and melatonin can be used with discretion. Maintaining a routine is highly essential, too. Late night snacking is harmful for health and for your sleep pattern.

Your body should not get any charge or trigger that hinders your sleep. If you suffer from sleep apnea or insomnia and home remedies are not working, then you must consult a professional for this purpose.

## Mindfulness and Its Role in Reducing Inflammation

Being Mindful is the opposite of being **"Mind Full"**. It is not just one less "l" but a life changer.

It means you are living in the present and are not judging what is happening right now. Everything just passes your mind. It involves high levels of focus in the time at hand.

Daily mindfulness practices include full body scans, deep breathing, meditation, mindful eating etc. Mindful eating means that you are fully involved with all the five senses in the food that you are eating.

Mindful lifestyle helps reduce stress and improves focus and provides a sense of achievement. It helps in reducing the chances of chronic inflammation. Imagine that you are eating anti-inflammatory ingredients such as nuts in your meal and doing that mindfully, it increases the benefits by two folds. Mindfulness is a mindset and does not require much effort once it becomes a routine.

A daily practice of as little as 5 minutes can help to begin with.

Answer your mindful practice questions right now and taste the benefits:

Name any five things around you that you can see

Name any four things around you that you can hear

Name any three things around your room that you can smell

Name any two things around you that you can feel

Name any one thing around you that you can taste (you may imagine a taste of any food)

Such practices can help you focus on the world around you and make you come out of your mind and loops of thoughts.

**Integrating Natural Supplements with Diet**

Natural supplements such as garlic, turmeric, herbs, spices, seeds, omega-3 supplements, and nuts can be added to the diet to supplement the anti-inflammatory properties. However, caution must be exercised for starting a new supplement, especially if you are taking some sort of medication or have a diagnosed health condition.

You must also look for a variety of supplements by alternating all varieties in order to avoid any excess or deficiencies. Monitor your symptoms of inflammation and general health such as joint and muscle fatigue, sleep patterns, headaches or any other common symptom that you face. Regular monitoring and maintaining a diary helps you see what remedies or supplements are improving your situation and which are not. Such diaries can be digitized for easy access from anywhere so that you don't have to take your hard cover diary everywhere. You just can take a picture and upload or save a small comment on your symptoms on apps even if not at home.

**Home Remedies to Enhance Anti-Inflammatory Benefits**

Other than the diets or supplements that have anti-inflammatory properties, home remedies such as using relaxation techniques of Epsom salt baths, using herbal teas, aroma therapy etc. have benefits in reducing stress. The food we consume has active ingredients that have antioxidant properties. Such ingredients are called phytochemicals and have several benefits including being anti-inflammatory.

However, remedies such as taking a warm water bath with Epsom salt helps increase blood circulation and increases the dilation of blood vessels for easy flow of blood. Blood carries food and oxygen for muscles and takes away the metabolites. Such remedies can be used at home but sometimes need professional advice, too. If the condition does not improve, you must immediately consult a relevant health expert to discuss your situation. An anti-inflammatory diet along with such home remedies do help in enhancing the overall potential of what you consume and helps to maintain a long-term healthy life.

# CHAPTER 8

## *The Sustainable Anti-Inflammatory Lifestyle*

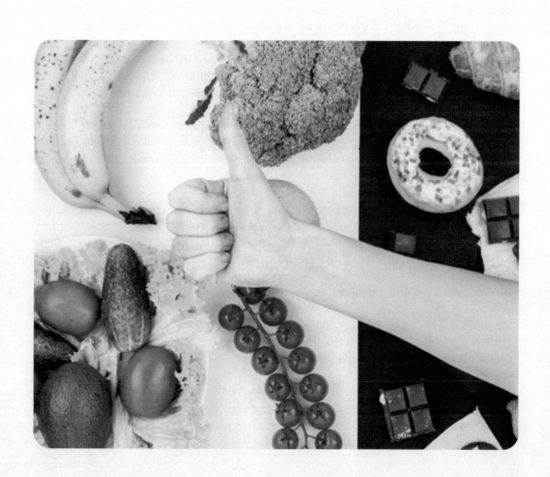

It is not a compulsion to eat everything right to follow an anti-inflammatory diet. You have to choose a long-term workable plan in which there is no feeling of being left out and allows you to enjoy your life along with additional benefits of an anti-inflammatory diet.

# Making Smart Choices When Dining Out

Although we always prefer home-made food items, eating away from home sometimes becomes a necessity. During those times, you need to be aware of what your choices are at a restaurant and ensure that those choices will help you in choosing and sticking to an anti-inflammatory dietary pattern.

Some ingredients and preparation methods contribute to the anti-inflammatory potential of a recipe. For instance, recipes which contain ingredients that are fried, processed, sugary, refined, high sodium etc. are not recommended for frequent use. Instead, recipes which are baked, grilled or sautéed instead of deep fried, less processed, contain whole grains, vegetables and fruits are more likely to have better anti-inflammatory potential.

You may look for specific phytonutrients rich ingredients in the recipe description while choosing from the menu. If the menu card does not contain enough information, you may request the waiter to ask the manager or chef to explain what major ingredients they put in their recipe.

Just like someone who has gluten intolerance would look for ingredients containing wheat in recipes (including the coating, marinades, thickeners), an anti-inflammatory diet must also be handled in a similar manner. Some pan Asian cuisine have a high usage of chillies and garlic, Turkish restaurants have a frequent use of grilled meat, cheese and tomatoes.

You may choose certain cuisine to reduce the chances of developing or exacerbating the inflammation. Avoid overeating at restaurants. Sometimes buffet service provides a large variety of food items from which to choose, but they also create a barrier in restricting oneself from overeating. You need to be deliberately out of such situations where overeating is likely to occur.

### Growing Your Own Anti-Inflammatory Ingredients

Home farming has many benefits and is great for people who love fresh, homegrown foods. Grow your own vegetables for fresher, better flavors, and added benefits. You can take control of your medications, go organic, and avoid harmful chemicals.

Beyond these obvious benefits, using your own homegrown produce brings a deep sense of satisfaction and makes every meal a personal success. Choose a sunny location, preferably one that gets at least six hours of direct sunlight. Start with easy-to-grow plants like herbs, greens, and tomatoes.

Herbs like basil and mint add fresh flavor to dishes, while leafy greens like spinach and kale are versatile and can be harvested multiple times. Tomatoes are a garden favorite and are perfect for many recipes.

Maximize space by using wall-mounted planters. Community gardens are another great option that provide shared land for people to grow their own vegetables and foster community connections.

Fresh herbs enhance the flavor of sauces and marinades, vegetables can be used in salads or smoothies, and tomatoes can be used in sauces, soups, or fresh salads. By using homemade products, you not only enjoy the best taste and nutrition, but you also get more satisfaction from your gardening activities.

## Preserving Seasonal Produce for Year-Round Use

Preserving food is an important skill that allows you to enjoy your produce outside of its growing season. You can choose from a variety of methods, each suitable for different types of produce. Freezing is ideal for fruits, vegetables, and herbs because it preserves their flavor and nutrients with minimal effort.

Drying, on the other hand, works well with herbs, tomatoes, and berries, focusing on their flavor and making them easy to store. Canning is an option for preserving many fruits, vegetables, and even meats, but careful attention to safety

procedures is required to prevent spoilage. Pickled produce retains most of its nutritional value and can provide important vitamins and antioxidants even when fresh options don't. This is especially useful in winter or in areas where there is no growing season, allowing you to get the best results from anti-inflammatory foods like tomatoes and greens.

To freeze produce, wash and cut the produce, blanch vegetables to preserve color and texture, and use airtight containers or bags. For drying, use a dehydrator or oven to dry produce evenly to prevent mold. For canning, sterilize jars, prepare produce, and put in sterilized cans.

Use frozen fruit in smoothies, dried herbs in soups and stews, and canned tomatoes in sauces and casseroles. Preserved ingredients not only enhance your meals, but they also encourage healthy food consumption all year round.

## Educating Others About Anti-Inflammatory Choices

Discussing the benefits of anti-inflammatory diets with friends and family should be thoughtful and respectful. Start by sharing your own experiences and the positive impact they have had on your health and well-being.

Use simple, relevant words and give examples of how a healthy diet can increase your energy levels or reduce pain. Share trusted resources or tips for working together to discover anti-inflammatory foods to make the discussion more productive. Use colorful fruits and vegetables and prepare them carefully to create filling, hearty meals. Give each dish a small label or description to highlight its health benefits and ingredients.

Consider offering a variety of options to accommodate different tastes and dietary preferences. This approach not only educates your guests, but also makes the meal more appealing to non-foodies. Consider writing a blog or article explaining the benefits of the diet, giving practical advice, and sharing delicious recipes. Social media platforms are also powerful tools; share content, engaging information, and personal success stories to reach an audience.

## Celebrating Your Success and Next Steps

Knowing what's important for your immune system is an important way to stay motivated and celebrate success. Whether you're celebrating a diet or noticing improvements in your health, these milestones can be central to your commitment and well-being. Consider keeping a journal or creating a visual diary to record and reflect on your accomplishments.

Taking this time to celebrate, even in small ways, will help fuel your passion and keep you passionate about life. When you reach your current goals, take the time to evaluate your progress and set new, higher but realistic goals. Choose healthy gifts that complement your lifestyle, like a spa vacation, investing in quality cooking equipment, or eating in a kitchen that explores new foods.

These rewards should align with your goals and provide motivation without compromising your commitment. Adjust your diet to meet your changing nutritional needs as you age and continue to seek out foods that support your health. Plan ahead by researching local stores when traveling.

When it comes to family strength, include loved ones in meal planning and support planning. By staying strong and resilient, you can maintain a healthy lifestyle and reap the benefits.

# Continuous Learning and Adaptation in Your Diet Journey

Keeping up-to-date with the latest research on anti-inflammatory diets is essential to improving your health. Knowledge about food is constantly evolving, and new research can provide insight into the effectiveness of different dietary strategies.

When you come across new research, evaluate how it fits your own needs. Education is an important part of health. Pay attention to how different foods and habits affect your body and energy. Adjust your diet based on what works best for you, including your personal preferences and health responses.

Remember, diet is important, but combining it with exercise, stress management, and good sleep is crucial for overall health. Take the first step to transform your health using the ideas in this book. Be patient and persistent as changing your diet takes time.

That is because you are not only changing your diet, you are changing your life. Share your success to inspire others and continue to learn and improve your approach. Experience the positive impact an immune-boosting lifestyle can have on your life and gain confidence in your ability to develop a healthy lifestyle.

# *References*

- Alam, W., Khan, H., Shah, M. A., Cauli, O., & Saso, L. (2020). Kaempferol as a dietary anti-inflammatory agent: current therapeutic standing. Molecules, 25(18), 4073.

- Banez, M. J., Geluz, M. I., Chandra, A., Hamdan, T., Biswas, O. S., Bryan, N. S., & Von Schwarz, E. R. (2020). A systemic review on the antioxidant and anti-inflammatory effects of resveratrol, curcumin, and dietary nitric oxide supplementation on human cardiovascular health. Nutrition Research, 78, 11-26.

- Campmans-Kuijpers, M. J., & Dijkstra, G. (2021). Food and food groups in inflammatory bowel disease (IBD): The design of the Groningen anti-inflammatory diet (GrAID). Nutrients, 13(4), 1067.

- Shahbazi, R., Sharifzad, F., Bagheri, R., Alsadi, N., Yasavoli-Sharahi, H., & Matar, C. (2021). Anti-inflammatory and immunomodulatory properties of fermented plant foods. Nutrients, 13(5), 1516.

- Wawrzyniak-Gramacka, E., Hertmanowska, N., Tylutka, A., Morawin, B., Wacka, E., Gutowicz, M., & Zembron-Lacny, A. (2021). The association of anti-inflammatory diet ingredients and lifestyle exercise with inflammation. Nutrients, 13(11), 3696.

## HASSLE FREE ANTİ-İNFLAMMATORY DİET COOKBOOK

HELP US GROW WİTH YOUR REVİEW!

**WE'D LOVE YOUR FEEDBACK!**

THANK YOU FOR CHOOSİNG THİS BOOK AS PART OF YOUR HEALTH JOURNEY. YOUR FEEDBACK MEANS THE WORLD TO US! IF YOU'VE ENJOYED THE RECİPES AND FOUND THE İNFORMATİON HELPFUL, PLEASE CONSİDER LEAVİNG A POSİTİVE REVİEW. SİMPLY SCAN THE QR CODE BELOW TO SHARE YOUR THOUGHTS.

YOUR REVİEW HELPS US REACH MORE PEOPLE AND CONTİNUE SPREADİNG THE MESSAGE OF HEALTHY LİVİNG.

## THANK YOU FOR YOUR SUPPORT!

# RECIPES INDEX

# RECIPES INDEX

Made in the USA
Columbia, SC
23 December 2024

50588339R00065